T0271468

'What struck me when I first read this book was the elegance of its words, the easy wisdom of the ideas expressed by its creator, and the beautiful blend of Eastern philosophies with the modern world that filled its pages... *Qigong in Yoga Teaching and Practice* will not only widen your horizons and open your heart, it will inspire you to deepen into yourself, to taste the beauty of life as it flows through you, and will likely help you to feel simply more energetic, and equally more calm at the same time. Highly recommended.'

– Judith Hanson Lasater, PhD, PT, yoga teacher and author
of ten books including Yoga Myths: What You Need to Learn
and Unlearn for a Safe and Happy Yoga Practice

'Joo Teoh's book is a pearl of universal wisdom, spoken from a deep well of penetrating insight. Highly recommended.'

– Max Strom, international breathing teacher and author of
A Life Worth Breathing *and* There is No APP for Happiness

'Here is a book which gives the reader a glimpse into what the world looks like through the lens of a profound, practical and insightful Chinese culture. How lyrical and rich the Chinese language is in describing our body, the meridians, nature and our relationships. With Joo's cultural experiences, growing up in Malaysia, a country with Chinese, Indian, British and Malay roots, having an education in the West and living in Malaysia, the USA, the UK, China and France with a practice of Traditional Chinese Medicine and yoga, what better person to describe and explain the philosophy of Qigong in the practice of Yoga.'

– Dr Marie Shieh, FRACGP, Anna Bay, NSW Australia

Yoga Teaching Guides

As it grows in popularity, teaching yoga requires an increasing set of skills and understanding, in terms of both yoga practice and knowledge. This series of books guides you towards becoming an accomplished, trusted yoga teacher by refining your teaching skills and methods. The series, written by experts in the field, focuses on the key topics for yoga teachers – including sequencing, language in class, anatomy and running a successful and thriving yoga business – and presents practical information in an accessible manner and format for all levels. Each book is filled with visual aids to enhance the reading experience, and includes 'top tips' to highlight and emphasise key ideas and advice.

in the same series

**Supporting Yoga Students with
Common Injuries and Conditions**
A Handbook for Teachers and Trainees
Andrew McGonigle
ISBN 978 1 78775 469 0
eISBN 978 1 78775 470 6

of related interest

Yoga Teaching Handbook
A Practical Guide for Yoga
Teachers and Trainees
Edited by Sian O'Neill
ISBN 978 1 84819 355 0
eISBN 978 0 85701 313 2

Daoist Meridian Yoga
Activating the Twelve Pathways for
Energy Balance and Healing
Camilo Sanchez, L.Ac., MOM
ISBN 978 1 84819 285 0
eISBN 978 0 85701 236 4

**Integrating Philosophy in
Yoga Teaching and Practice**
A Practical Guide
Wendy Teasdill
ISBN 978 1 78775 135 4
eISBN 978 1 78775 136 1

QIGONG IN YOGA TEACHING AND PRACTICE

Understanding Qi and the
Use of Meridian Energy

Joo Teoh

Foreword by Mimi Kuo-Deemer
Series Editor: Sian O'Neill

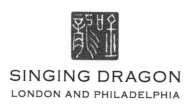

SINGING DRAGON
LONDON AND PHILADELPHIA

First published in Great Britain in 2021 by Singing Dragon,
an imprint of Jessica Kingsley Publishers
An Hachette Company

1

Copyright © Joo Teoh 2021

The right of Joo Teoh to be identified as the Author of the Work has been asserted
by him in accordance with the Copyright, Designs and Patents Act 1988.

Foreword copyright © Mimi Kuo-Deemer 2021
Photographs copyright © Joo Teoh and Patrick Ardagh-Walter 2021

All rights reserved. No part of this publication may be reproduced, stored in a retrieval system,
or transmitted, in any form or by any means without the prior written permission of the
publisher, nor be otherwise circulated in any form of binding or cover other than that in which
it is published and without a similar condition being imposed on the subsequent purchaser.

A CIP catalogue record for this title is available from the
British Library and the Library of Congress

ISBN 978 1 78775 652 6
eISBN 978 1 78775 653 3

Printed and bound in Great Britain by CPI Group

Jessica Kingsley Publishers' policy is to use papers that are natural, renewable and recyclable
products and made from wood grown in sustainable forests. The logging and manufacturing
processes are expected to conform to the environmental regulations of the country of origin.

Jessica Kingsley Publishers
Carmelite House
50 Victoria Embankment
London EC4Y 0DZ

www.singingdragon.com

This book is dedicated to my Beijing Family.

CONTENTS

Foreword by Mimi Kuo-Deemer   9

Acknowledgements   12

Preface   13

1. Shape and No Shape   17
   Ethics and intention   19
   The heart of qigong   20
   Moving naturally and freely   21

2. Cultivating Qi   26
   Breathing the breath   28
   'Ma shang lai!'   30
   Horse Stance   31
   Qualities of qi and dynamics of movement   32

3. The Qi Circulatory System   40
   Part 1: The central meridians   40
   Part 2: The Emperor and his Ministers   48

4. Exercises to Stimulate the Meridians   55
   Heart meridian   55
   Small Intestine meridian   60
   Bladder meridian   63
   Kidney meridian   65
   Pericardium meridian   73

Triple Heater meridian 75

Liver and Gallbladder meridians 79

Lung meridian 81

Large Intestine meridian 88

Stomach and Spleen meridians 92

5. Bringing Qi to the Arms and Legs 97

Part 1: Building qi in the hands and arms 97

Part 2: Moving qi to the legs 107

6. Inspirations for Sequencing 112

Part 1: The Five Elements 112

Part 2: Seasonal transitions 123

Part 3: Pairing meridians 128

Part 4: Inspiration from Chinese herbalism 133

Postscript 136

Glossary of Chinese Terms and Pronunciation Guide 138

Further Study 149

Subject Index 151

Index of Exercises 155

Index of Yoga Poses for Sequencing,
Transitions and Variations 156

Index of Acupuncture Point Names in English 158

FOREWORD

I first met Joo in a yoga studio in Beijing, China in 2006. He had come to take class at Yoga Yard, a studio founded by myself and a fellow American, Robyn Wexler. It did not take long before Joo became one of the studio's most beloved teachers, as well as an enduring friend. He taught what many teachers at Yoga Yard drew on: yoga influenced by qigong and theories underlying Chinese medicine. *Qigong in Yoga Teaching and Practice* is the accumulated experience of Joo's more than 15 years of study, exploration and dedication to two rich and evolving traditions of yoga and qigong.

While most people in the world today have been exposed to yoga and know what it is, far fewer have come across qigong. The reasons for this are layered. One reason is the relatively limited exchange of ideas between China and the West – especially compared with that which took place between India and the West. With India's steady ties to Britain in its colonial and postcolonial eras, exchange flourished, whereas in the wake of China's civil wars and victory of Chairman Mao's Chinese Communist Party in 1949, China closed itself off to the outside. It was not until economic reforms began in 1979 that a growing number of China's cultural traditions, from Classical Chinese Medicine to martial arts, started to flow into the mainstream of Western society. A second reason has to do with yoga's more successful worldwide marketing compared with qigong: think of slim, youthful images of people in a yoga handstand at the beach, versus someone pictured standing in qigong's foundational posture, *Wuji*, with their arms rounded in front of their chest, clad in baggy silk pyjamas! And finally, qigong is like moving meditation: practices tend to be slower and rarely induce a sweat. Like any approach to Chinese medicine, it works gradually, creating deeper, lasting shifts in our organ and meridian systems. Anything that takes time and patience is a harder sell in our modern world, where people strive to express mail themselves across the finish line to a healthier, happier life.

Fortunately, times are changing. More people today are discovering qigong's subtle yet powerful and transformative ability to rebalance energy and foster vibrant health. Among many yoga teachers and dedicated students, interest in qigong has blossomed into a particularly strong affinity. This comes as no surprise, especially given the popularity of Yin Yoga and an ever-growing number of yoga teacher trainings that include approaches to how Traditional Chinese Medicine can be applied to yoga practice. Rather than diluting the tradition, I believe this integrative approach expands and enriches the experience and embodiment of yoga. Also, a yoga practice imbued with qigong's imagery of the natural world can impact the way we experience and relate to our environment. The emphasis on observing and learning about nature's balance and harmony in qigong comes at a time when our species and the fate of our planet face a dire and ecologically disastrous future. We are part of nature manifest in human form. When we recognise this, we start to see that when we take care of ourselves, we are taking care of our planet.

Yoga and qigong are living traditions that continually evolve and grow. When we attempt to keep traditions from changing and cling to a sense of ownership, we start to erect boundaries and strict ideas of right and wrong. This is a human tendency. Yet, if one definition of yoga is the expansion of consciousness and a path to liberation, or *mokṣa*, then the orientation and evolution of practice can also be seen as what liberates us from rigid beliefs and narrowing, confining orthodoxies.

In the world we inhabit today, attempts to prove accuracy over fallacy have polarised our political as well as social realms to the point where basic rights and freedoms are endangered. Any willingness to bridge and build commonality between cultures and practices comes as a relief. By bringing together yoga and qigong, yoga teachers and students can not only gain new insights into how they approach their practice and health, but also discover ways to inject positive value and innovation into the inevitable dialectic of change.

As an acupuncturist, yoga teacher and qigong teacher, Joo is a pioneer at the frontier of an exciting and evolving point in history where ancient traditions can meld together. In this unique book with an equally unique voice, he grants a refreshing space to his readers to explore, adapt and reshape the way we can structure and approach yoga and qigong. Part of his ability to share this progressive approach stems from his ability to defy conventional definitions of culture and identity. As an ethnically Chinese man who grew up in Malaysia, was schooled in the UK and lived and worked in the US and China, he is uniquely positioned to move between cultures and fuse the best of them together. As a trained acupuncturist, he also offers a deeper understanding of the theories behind Chinese medicine's laws of association, balance and treatment.

Qigong in Yoga Teaching and Practice is a book that navigates two ancient systems of mental, physical and spiritual discipline beautifully. It offers a rich resource and guide into the theories behind Chinese medicine that underlie qigong forms, as well as practical examples of class themes and sequences based on the Chinese Five Elements to get you started. Whether you are a yoga teacher interested in deepening your understanding of Chinese medicine, or a teacher keen to start mixing qigong forms into your yoga asana classes, this book will offer you a treasure trove of insights and possibilities to grow your practice, teaching and love of yoga.

Mimi Kuo-Deemer, author of
Qigong and the Tai Chi Axis and *Xiu Yang*

ACKNOWLEDGEMENTS

To my teachers Cameron Tukapua, Matthew Raymond Cohen, Max Strom, Judith Hanson Lasater, Donna Farhi, Sarah Powers and Gerad Kite, thank you for sharing your rich knowledge, for your enduring dedication and your generous guidance.

To Mimi Kuo-Deemer, thank you for being an inspiration and for believing in me.

To Patrick Ardagh-Walter, your help with this book has been invaluable. Thank you for your generosity, curiosity, time and faith in me.

To Martina Merlet, Silja Frey and Anne Wang, thank you for reading the early drafts, for your encouragement and for your sisterhood.

To Mum, Pa and Zhen, thank you for believing in me. I love you.

To Sian O'Neill, thank you for your guidance, patience and trust throughout this process.

To Sarah Hamlin and the team at Singing Dragon, thank you for your enthusiasm, responsiveness and generous support.

To every single one of my students, past and present, thank you. You have taught me more than you will ever know.

This book was written under lockdown, while I was recovering from COVID-19. I send my deepest gratitude to my new family, friends and students here in la Manche for their support and love during this time. Mes ami(e)s Manchois(es), je vous remercie pour vos encouragements et votre soutien. Au plaisir de se retrouver au bord de la mer, au tapis, sur scène, et aux repas.

PREFACE

In 2006, while living in Beijing, I hit a plateau in my yoga practice. I was doing strong 90-minute vinyasa classes four or five times a week, and instead of feeling energised, I felt drained by the practice. I spoke to my teacher at the time, Mimi, who suggested that I attend some workshops with a teacher visiting from Los Angeles. 'His name is Matthew and he does this cool thing where he mixes tai chi and yoga,' Mimi told me. Not only did I do four of his workshops, I also found myself on my first teacher training course with Matthew Raymond Cohen a few months later. That year, I also met Cameron Tukapua, a wise woman and experienced healer, an acupuncturist, founder of Christchurch College of Holistic Healing and teacher of Traditional Chinese Medicine. She revealed to me a much deeper understanding of the Five Elements, which in turn led to my study with Gerad Kite, founder of the London Institute of Five Element Acupuncture. Along with Mimi, Matthew, Cameron and Gerad, I am very grateful and fortunate to also call Max Strom and Judith Hanson Lasater my teachers. Their honesty, their humour, their knowledge and their humanity still guide the way I teach and practise today.

Since incorporating qigong into my daily life and yoga practice, my physical practice no longer exhausts me. I believe deeply in the healing potential of blending yoga and qigong. It is what I practise, and it is what I have been teaching since 2007. My practice consists of clear intention, strong breath, flowing movement and conscious rest. The exercises are drawn from yoga asana, *pranayama*, mudra, mantra, Daoist teachings, Chinese medicine and acupuncture, qigong and the Five Elements. In this

book I want to inspire you to explore the practice of qigong and to incorporate its principles, exercises and themes into your yoga.

Chinese medicine and acupuncture have greatly influenced my
qigong and my yoga. When I learnt that each acupuncture point has its
own spirit, its own properties and uses, my whole universe expanded. It
will take several lifetimes to understand every single one of these points,
but I am daring to share what I have grasped so far. You do not have to
read and write Chinese to appreciate the meaning of a Chinese phrase.
Similarly, you do not need to be a licensed acupuncturist to accurately
locate an acupuncture point.

Hanyu Pinyin names are used for acupuncture points throughout this
book because the English names differ in various traditions of acupuncture. The pronunciation guide provided in the Glossary should help you
navigate the names without needing the fundamentals of Chinese tones.
Should I fail to guide you to the location of any point, search the reference
numbers for the point on the internet. These are more consistent (but not
identical) across different styles of acupuncture.

Awareness of Chinese medicine gives greater depth to each exercise.
The meanings behind meridians and points are simple to understand
because they arise from the observation of nature. Why reinvent the wheel
when we already understand everything there is to learn? Yet, I am wary
because 'a little learning is a dang'rous thing'.

- This book does not go into the origins and history of qigong, nor
  does it compare yoga philosophy with Daoism. My recommended
  texts are listed in the Further Study section.

- While thousands of exercises use the term qigong (and none of them
  are wrong to do so), this book contains instructions for only 60.

- While the twelve primary meridian lines are fairly consistent across
  different styles of acupuncture, I have not indicated all meridian
  lines, only the fourteen most commonly used. The Conception
  Vessel and Governor Vessel are often included within a category
  called Eight Extraordinary Meridians.

- Traditional Chinese Medicine was taught differently before and
  after the formation of the People's Republic of China. Be aware

that this could be a reason for any differences in what you read here and elsewhere.

- The Five Elements are also known as, amongst other things, the Five Phases, Five Movements, Five Ways, Five Stages, Five Agents, Five Poisons and Five Virtues.

What I am confident of is this: there are no absolutes in the expression and interpretation of the theory and practice. My interpretation and expression here in this book will jar with some practitioners: this tension is necessary and fruitful. Our incomplete knowledge is fertile ground for new growth. This is the way of the Dao: there is room for all of us. My suggestions for further study demonstrate, I hope, the strength that comes from diversity.

No two people ever make a cake the exact same way: my husband follows a recipe to the gram, whereas I am much less precise. Nevertheless, we both bake delicious cakes. Most of us approach practice and teaching somewhere along this spectrum, with a balance of clear instruction and adequate room to freestyle. In this book you will find building blocks to experiment with and incorporate into your own practices, and then eventually into your classes. Many of these are complete practices within themselves, which you can string together to make a sequence, examples of which you will find in Chapter 6. I encourage you to take your time, to understand how these exercises feel in your body and to play with them until they appear in a sequence that is authentically yours. This will give you confidence to express, in your own way, the subtleties and nuances.

When we go against nature, we suffer. When we allow ourselves to synchronise with the rhythms surrounding us, we flow and grow with ease. This is what I want to share. Not everything here will land at first reading, so keep exploring, keep experimenting and trust that you will find your own flow. In this polarised and competitive world, qigong offers us a way to find harmony with our surroundings and be at ease in our body. My wish is for qigong to bring you some refreshment.

Joo Chye Teoh
Soulles, France
October 2020

Chapter 1

SHAPE AND NO SHAPE

*Jing, Qi and Shen, those of no shape. Tendons, bones
and flesh, those with shape. The method is to train those
with shape to be the collaborators of those with no shape.
Cultivate those with no shape as assistants of those
with shape. It is one but two, and is two but one.*
YI JIN JING (MUSCLE/TENDON CHANGE CLASSIC) CIRCA 502 CE

Three important elements, called the Three Treasures, in qigong are the *jing*, meaning vital essence, the qi, meaning energy, and the *shen*, the spirit. These are the intangible components of life. *Jing* creates life, qi powers life and *shen* gives meaning to life. Our vital essence, our *jing*, is inherited from the interaction of cells and genetic material at our conception. According to Chinese medicine, this essence is stored within our kidneys and powers our growth through life. The energy we take in through daily nourishment via the lungs and stomach is a daily top-up of vital essences, like rain falling on a reservoir. This top-up is different from natural flow from the source, be it a spring or the rivers that formed the reservoir in the first place, because it will never fill the reservoir as much as the source does.

Regarding shape and no shape, the passage above goes on to say that it is futile to cultivate one more than the other, or to pitch one against the other. Their relationship is mutual, not dependent. Giving equal attention to both will result in a strong body in which the tangible and intangible are united.

The combustion and consumption of the nourishment within us is what makes qi. This is the energy available to us to live our lives. It circulates in the body through our blood, it is believed, which is why the blood pulse is central to Chinese medicine. The way we manage our physical body directly affects our ability to generate qi, and qigong therefore has a rich variety of physical exercises designed to maintain the physical health of the internal organs. The internal organs do the work of processing and transforming nourishment into qi. This includes the management of detritus and the necessary elimination that comes with the process of combustion. Eleven organs are identified and assigned importance: the heart, the pericardium, the bladder, the kidneys, the lungs, the small and large intestines, the liver, the gallbladder, the stomach and the spleen. There is a 12th, which has a function but no form, called the Triple Heater. The Chinese see the Triple Heater as a system of regulating warmth within the torso, which is divided into three spaces where nourishment is received, cooked and transformed into qi.

Shen means spirit; but what is captured in the Chinese character indicates much more. The character for *shen* is drawn as the sun, sky, day and moon with two hands on a rope. This depicts *shen* as an on-going process of understanding the divine machinations of mortal life. It is not clear whether the hands are pulling the rope, climbing the rope or trying to unknot it, but the strokes indicate humans interacting with divinity. Our spirits are changeable from day to day, moment to moment, but the English word 'spirit' tends to confine the concept to a sole object, ethereal though this object may be. *Shen* is divinity expressed as the *je ne sais quoi*, the sparkle in our eyes, the wind beneath our wings, the fizz, the pizazz, the laugh, the hug, the lightbulb moment, or the faith to endure. *Shen* is the tangible yet unknown that carries us through the activity of mortal life.

In the *Huangdi Neijing*, the foundation text for Chinese medicine, the depressed Emperor asks his Minister a series of questions, seeking to understand his afflictions and state of dis-ease. 'Where does this state come from? Should we accuse heaven? Or is it the fault of human kind?' He is desperate to assign responsibility to himself – either for having gone astray or for having failed to rise to the challenge that heaven presented to him. He goes on, 'And what are virtue, qi, life, essences, spirits, *hun, po,* heart, intent, will, thought, wisdom, and reflection? Please instruct me in this.' His Minister answers, 'Heaven within me is virtue, earth within me is qi.'[1] Following the lead in the wise Minister's reply, we approach our qigong practice first with the divine, and then we work with the manifest.

If we remove the Chinese words from the quote above, it seems strikingly aligned with the aim of a yoga practice, where we use the body to calm the mind. These two traditions have complementary values and virtues too vast to be contained in one volume. This book will focus on some useful aspects of movement that blend well with the flow of yoga asana. It will also introduce the core principles and values carried by this rich and still-evolving practice.

Ethics and intention

The Emperor's Minister continues in his answer, 'Virtue flows, qi spreads out, and there is life.' The conscious choices we make are expressions of our ethics. These ethics are the values we hold in life; these are the virtues we strive to live by. They are present in our interactions with our students. They are present in the intentions we bring into a teaching space. As teachers living in a multicultural, multilingual world, we must be mindful of our language and the implications of any words we use. It is increasingly easy to be misunderstood. It is increasingly easy to offend unintentionally. It is therefore important to be specific and to be clear. Here are some ethical qualities or virtues that are consistent in all faiths, all cultures and all geographies, and which can be understood in all languages in the world:

- Kindness

- Discipline

- Gratitude

- Respect

- Mindfulness

---

1   Larre, C. and Rochat de la Vallée, E. (1991) *The Heart: In Ling Shu Chapter 8.* Cambridge: Monkey Press.

- Honesty

- Responsibility

- Virtuous sexuality

- Voluntary simplicity

- Contentment

- Study

- Humility.

I was first introduced to this way of looking at ethics by Max Strom, and I maintain his practice of using non-dogmatic language in my classes. I encourage you to make your own list of virtues or ethical values, and to express in your own words what they mean for you and the actions you take to practise them in daily life. These can become enduring and compelling points of departure for your professional and personal growth as a teacher, or, specifically, for creating a theme for one class.

Two idioms often quoted in qigong teaching are '*Yong yi, bu yong li*' and '*You yi, you qi, you li.*' The first phrase means 'Use intention, do not use force,' and the second phrase means 'Have intention, have energy, have strength.' In both these idioms, intention comes first. The Chinese character for intention, *yi*, is made of two components: sound and heart. Intent is what resonates from the heart. To go further, the components that make up the character for sound are characters *li*, which means to stand or to establish, and *ri*, which means the sun or the day. These elements condense into a sense of immediacy within the word *yi*: within our hearts, where do we stand at this moment in time? Start here. Start with clear, simple intention, formed from the values you hold dear in your heart.

The heart of qigong

Motion and dedication lie at the heart of qigong. The traditional Chinese characters for the words qi and *gong* indicate how continuous movement, and momentum, must be maintained in order for any effort to yield useful results. The character for qi in traditional Chinese writing indicates energy generated by the combustion of grain as food. Sitting above this part of the character are strokes meaning the rising up of vapours, a moment that is ephemeral. In contemporary daily life, the word qi means breath, energy, life force, spirit. The character for *gong* comprises a component meaning work, labour, craft or skill, and another meaning strength, power or force. The word *gong* on its own is commonly used to mean achievement or merit, success attained via skilful effort. In this book, *qigong* refers to the expressions of effort and discipline used to generate immediate vitality through the transformation of alimentation (fuel) into energy (rising vapours). Continuous effort must be maintained should a steady stream of energy be desired. In short, skilful toil yields merit.

In qigong, the matter with which we toil is anything we allow into our breath, into our body and into our mind. The taking in is inevitable: to live, we must breathe, we must eat, we must drink, we must communicate and be in relationship to our surroundings. How skilfully our body, mind and breath transform these inputs into useful outcomes is influenced by how we maintain a healthy functioning body, a clear mind and steady breath, and equally by the quality of the input. This is why the practices and ideas presented in qigong are framed as measures to correct an imbalance, or as a means to improve the health or function of specific elements of our being in anticipation of future austerity.

Moving naturally and freely

Pause for a moment right now and imagine a beautiful person walking into the room and sitting down beside you. Imagine this person is naked. Now, imagine this person is a child. Imagine this child is crying. Notice how, in three or four seconds, your mental, emotional, maybe even physical sensations have changed. Another example: reach out both arms. Imagine holding a ten-kilogram bag of rice in your left hand and a stick of cotton candy in your right hand. Notice not only how each arm may have responded differently to this suggestion, but also any other emotional or visual responses. You may still be wondering what the naked, crying child is doing.

As we work our body during yoga or qigong, as we give or respond to a verbal or physical instruction to move a certain way, there is no way to predict a set outcome or exact expression within our own body, and even less to expect one from our students. To begin moving naturally and freely, we must first avoid any temptation to organise or categorise what is inherently at once both chaotic and perfect: the full expression of life. Our first task is to get acquainted with the machinations of our own mind and body, and take responsibility for our habits.

The principles taught and practised in qigong can be learnt by observing and learning about nature, including human behaviour. This is true of the philosophy and also of its application to physical movement. Many postures and movements in qigong are named after things that happen in nature: movements of animals (e.g. Sparrowhawk Takes Flight), references to the stars and planets (e.g. Turn to Look at the Moon), the elements of nature (e.g. Pushing Waves), movements of plants (e.g. Willows Bending in the Wind), actions of humans (e.g. Mischievous Boy Kicks His Leg). While these are romantic and evocative, they also immediately indicate the trajectory and impulse involved in the movement. If we wish to deepen our understanding of these practices, and to move beyond them being mere physical exercise, we will benefit from examining more closely the ways in which nature really behaves.

You may have heard yoga teachers use phrases such as 'be like young bamboo', 'embody the qualities of water' or 'root down'. I certainly have used these words myself in the past. These phrases are often favoured because they quickly evoke simple, relatable imagery. However, what is suggested is not the full picture, is not the entire context and is not necessarily a reflection of what truly happens in nature. While we are somewhat limited by popular use of language, we owe ourselves the time and effort to discover what happens in nature and how it is reflected and replicated within us. We also owe our students this consideration and precision.

For example, the qualities suggested by the words 'young' and 'bamboo' may quickly stimulate a response implying youthfulness, strength, virility and flexibility, and can be a sufficient shortcut in a busy class. But, in honesty, how much time have we spent watching, touching, even growing some bamboo? Bamboo spikes emerge as tough, tight, segmented cones. In spring, they push up quickly, some varieties growing as much as one metre per day. This cone grows to become the trunk of the bamboo, in sections called culms, and sheds the outer layer as it gets taller and matures. The stems and leaves push through only when the culms reach a certain height. If, at any point during this process, the shoot was to be torn or damaged, the entire season's growth would be compromised. So, in fact, the primary qualities displayed by young bamboo are speed, single-mindedness in its growth and vulnerability.

While roots do grow downward, what gives trees, shrubs and other plants more stability are their horizontal roots that grip the earth around the plant. These outward roots grip the earth in every direction, covering a much wider area than the taproot, which is the single main root that goes down vertically. Stability is provided by the radiating spread of the root system horizontally, diagonally *and* down. A weed that grows freely in my garden is the flatweed or cat's-ear (*Hypochaeris radicata*). Flatweed has a stem that can grow up to 40cm tall, but its taproot only goes about five or six centimetres into the ground. The plant gets its strength and stability from its leaves, which grow at the base of the plant. These leaves grow as much as 15cm in length, opening out flat against the earth (hence its name) to provide a wide base for the stems to ascend from. Each time I remove a larger one, I am surprised about how much grip these leaves – not the root – have against the earth beneath. The DIY enthusiasts among you may be familiar with a screw-retaining plug for plasterboard walls, which was designed on the same principle. So when we use the word 'root' as a reference in nature to provide instruction, which aspect of behaviour or direction of movement are we asking our students to mimic? Instead of 'root down' do we actually mean 'widen the feet'?

We may use phrases such as 'move like water' or 'move like air'. How aware are we at any given moment that most of our body is made up of liquid? We know it, intellectually, but it is not something that our senses are designed to indicate until we are dehydrated. It is not a thought that most of us carry consciously in daily life. We *are* moving liquid each time we shift our gaze, or each time we raise a finger. Moreover, water particles contain gaseous elements. Gases are absorbed into the blood and transported throughout the body. So we *are* moving air, too. We just can't *feel* most of it.

The way we move depends entirely on what we are moving. Our experience of a movement practice like qigong requires an awareness of where we are starting from at any given point in time. We can start with any emotional or physical needs: we may need to release stress; we may need to replenish depleted energy levels; we may need to relieve a tight lower back; we may want to heal a broken heart or a weakened digestive system. Within the lack that drives our motivation towards a practice like qigong lies the humble jewel of what is unknown and unknowable.

If we pause often enough to acknowledge that our data sets are never complete and perfect, that our senses are simply not designed to capture or contain knowledge of everything we are doing, we may over time be able to embrace humility and be comfortable with our imperfect sensory perception.

We have a good amount of language for what we call 'the known', yet many of us often struggle to accept what remains unknown. We can only use our imperfect and incomplete data sets as a point of departure and make discoveries along the way. This holds true for practitioners and even more for teachers. We will not ever know the complete experience of being us, so let us never imply or pretend we can tell our students what to feel or how to be.

Provide instead a point of reference: our eternally forgiving planet Earth and her manifestations. Learn the ways she expresses herself. See ourselves in her motions, see ourselves moving with her, as part of her great mystery and beauty. Our moving bodies, our ever-changing minds, our fluctuating emotions are woven into the shifting fabric of all expressions of nature. As we move our flesh, blood, skin and bones, we sink, rise, turn, warm and cool as part of nature.

We can equally embrace that which is known and that which is unknown, and participate in the chaos of existing on this planet with a willingness to be who we are, where we are.

When we allow ourselves this luxury, we open ourselves to the wonder of our interconnectedness to the subtle magic that surrounds us: the morning dew that evaporates upon the touch of sunshine; the tree branch that does not resist the landing of a pigeon; the ocean dancing and flirting with the sand; the invisible earth that is compressed into gleaming jewels beneath our feet.

So, here is an exercise you can do before you step onto your mat at home or walk into a class to start teaching. Answer these questions as simply and honestly as you can:

- Where am I stable right now?

- In what aspect of my life am I flexible?

- Where could I potentially be a little less rigid?

- What would break me?

- Where do I hide when life hits me hard?

- What is in my secret fortress? Who would I let in?

- What unleashes joy within me?

- How has sadness rusted my heart?

- How do I care for myself or another?

- What is most valuable right now?

Our answers will change each time we revisit these questions. Add your own questions to the list. Do not pin life choices to any one answer. What matters is to ask ourselves the questions frequently, and to keep exploring the answers. As we toil for merit, the answers to these questions provide fuel for our growth.

— *Chapter 2* —

CULTIVATING QI

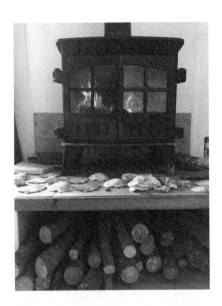 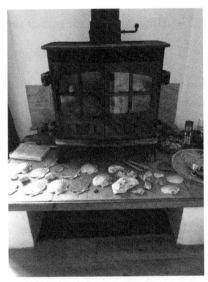

Compare these two photographs of the wood-burning stove in my kitchen. The visible differences are obvious, but contemplate what you may feel while looking at each of these images. In the first image, the wood store is full of logs, the fire is roaring healthily. In the second image, the wood store is empty, the embers are barely glowing. Between these two extremes there are, of course, many other stages, but this is a simple way to look at the benefit of a qigong practice: it is like being fully stocked in order to keep the fire of life burning. What matters is the preparation that leads to having a warm, lively fire burning in the stove. Filling the stove and lighting the wood is the easiest part of a process which, in actual fact, takes years of preparation.

We have a log store outdoors where our supply of firewood is stacked and kept dry throughout the winter. Whenever the indoor supply runs low, we bring in enough to fill the storage shelves for each of our three fireplaces. The stoves we have are of different sizes, the one in the kitchen being the smallest, so we stack the wood by size in the log store. This way, we know where to restock from when needed. Apart from one or two species of wood that can be burned 'green' or freshly cut, most wood needs to be stored and dried before it can be chopped to length, split and stacked. This is called seasoning the wood. Most wood that is cut in the spring time is seasoned for use over the following winter. Many people season their wood for much longer – two or three years – to remove as much moisture as possible, so that the wood burns better.

The supply of wood is also planned, with trees of different ages being coppiced or felled according to what is needed or when the tree is ready. Trees can be coppiced for wood from four years onwards. These stumps are then left to regrow for the next round of coppicing. Ample time and regular nourishment of the trees are therefore also required to ensure a future supply of firewood. Cut the tree too early, and you won't get much wood. It may even weaken the tree for subsequent growth. The quantity of fuel needed each winter will determine the number of trees being rotated for cutting. I won't go into further detail, but the message is clear, I hope. What we use in daily life – the dried wood – is the product of a longer process of planning and a chain of preparations.

Trees, being what they are, grow slowly. Many forests are planted generations ahead of their anticipated use. The same is true of the way in which we cultivate our qi for our current life: the energy we have for reproduction, the energy passed to offspring, these are a direct result of what we build up within ourselves to give. That with which we are born is naturally a result of what was passed from our parents, and to them from theirs. While we cannot change our ancestry, we can prepare for today and also for our future. How you choose to expend your energy is entirely your choice and responsibility. This commitment to work at it – the *gong* in qigong – means precisely that. This is the toil.

We replenish our stock of some resources for immediate consumption, while we cultivate some others and store them for use in the future, even when we do not feel an immediate lack. The practice of qigong is not intended as a strategy to manage fatigue. We can regularly stock up on qi reserves by consciously building and storing energy even when we do not need it. Unlike the log store outside my kitchen, we do not run out of 'storage space' for qi in our body. This is because simply living consumes qi. When a tree is planted for firewood, no one knows whose family room it will heat one day. When we perform exercises to replenish our energy reserves, we do so without any expectation of how and when we will need to expend them.

Breathing the breath

In Chinese, the noun for 'breath' and the verb meaning 'to breathe' are both *huxi*. *Huxi* translates as 'exhale inhale'. The Chinese verbs for 'to inhale', *xiqi*, and 'to exhale', *huqi*, use the same word for qi used in qigong. Breath is energy. What we take in with every inhalation and send out through each exhalation is energy. It does seem surprising, given how enmeshed breath and energy are in the Chinese language, that qigong is not known for its breathing practices in the way that *pranayama* is within yoga.

We will not go into specific qigong breathing exercises in this book. You will find exercises that are frequently taught in qigong schools for regulating the breath, called *tiao xi*, found in books by Dr Yang Jwing-Ming and *The Way of Qigong: The Art and Science of Chinese Energy Healing* by Kenneth S. Cohen (listed in the Further Study section).

For the exercises contained in this book, all we want is a steady, conscious breath. Breathe as naturally as you can, without straining, without striving. This is particularly important during exercises where a particularly slow movement has been accorded an inhale or exhale. If it becomes too challenging to breathe slowly, simply breathe naturally and freely, but continue to move the body slowly.

We all have to start where we are, within the body and habits that are ours. There is no point instructing a beginner on all the muscles involved in the process of one inhale and exhale if they have only recently learnt where the diaphragm is located. Over time, with practice, with increased awareness of one's individual physical circumstances and habits, a student can start to explore the capacity and willingness to stretch or challenge the breathing patterns that are 'normal' for them.

Our bodies and brains have conscious intelligence and reflexes to ensure that the body is not deprived of oxygen. As a yoga teacher, it is safe to assume that most people in class will be fit enough for aerobic exercise. Anyone with bronchitis or pneumonia is unlikely to be attending your class for the first time at the peak of illness, but do ask if your students have less evident conditions, such as sleep apnoea, asthma, chronic obstructive pulmonary disease, emphysema or cystic fibrosis. These conditions may affect the way that they inhale and exhale while moving their body, and their capacity to change the volume or duration of each breath. More importantly, this knowledge gives you, as the person leading the practice, an indication of where their mental or physical priorities may lie. For someone who already has breathing difficulties in daily life, it may grate to be instructed to 'pay more attention to your breath'.

To encourage students to prioritise their breathing, use phrases that help them to build awareness of their breath and influence the quality of their breathing. Use instructions like these:

- 'Where do you feel your breath in your body at this moment?'

- 'Breathe out as much as you can, but don't force it so far that you feel the need to gasp for air.'

- 'Let the breath come in naturally without sucking or pulling it in.'

- 'Remember to keep breathing. Do not hold your breath.'

- 'Keep your breath smooth and steady.'

- 'Relax your shoulders. Relax your belly. Perhaps find a smile. Notice how your breathing has changed.'

Health comes when qi can flow. An unobstructed canal is only useful if there is water flowing through it. The benevolence of our living body obliges the optimal transportation of oxygen to every body function and organ that requires it. Conscious, steady, easy breathing will encourage the student to take in more qi through the lungs, stimulate the heart to pump oxygenated blood, foster an awareness of breathing and develop an appreciation for each breath.

'Ma shang lai!'

When I was living and working in China, one of my daily frustrations was the lack of punctuality, or the inability of many people to commit to a timeframe for getting something done. This was true of travel visa bureaucracy, of making a transaction at the bank and even just of waiting for an order in a restaurant. The standard response when pressed for an update would be 'Ma shang lai! Ma shang lai!' or 'It's coming! It's coming!' The words used in the phrase are 'horse' (ma), 'up' (shang) and 'come' (lai). The expression means 'It is on the horse, it is on its way.' Dating back to the days of horseback messengers, the expression is evocative, simple to understand, but utterly and deliberately imprecise. It was all that was ever offered as salve for my impatience. Defeated, often I would mumble to myself in response 'Zhe pi ma zai na li ne?' – 'Where exactly is this blooming horse of yours, then?'

I tell this story for two reasons: first, because anyone can start a qigong practice at any stage of life. Simply start where you are, and do what you can. You don't need to carve out an hour every day to 'do it properly'. Five or ten minutes a day, every day, will do magic. You don't need to find a Shaolin temple or a Chinese master to start your practice. There are many good videos online that are available for free. Try various options until you find one that suits you. You may find subsequently that your motivation for finding a local teacher has changed.

The second reason is because in qigong practice, the posture of Horse Stance is often used as a starting posture for standing exercises. The way that the expression 'Ma shang lai!' is used in Chinese reminds me that there is aliveness to this posture as we imagine ourselves poised on horseback, on our way somewhere. There is immediacy but not urgency: our legs are positioned wider than usual, our spine is actively lengthening up, our feet are pressing down. It is a posture in which we are constantly working to stay stable. In Horse Stance, we want to concentrate stability in the centre of the body. At the same time, we want to anchor down through the feet and reach up through the crown of the head.

Horse Stance

This pose comes alive with subtlety and sensitivity. I never teach this pose in great detail at the start of a class. As I start a class, I simply instruct my students to stand comfortably, with the feet apart and stable. Only at the end of a session, when I have brought students back to quiet, do I invite sensitivity to the spaciousness and ease of this pose. Having said that, Horse Stance is a cornerstone and foundation of all movements, so I shall teach it now.

Stand comfortably. This is important. Comfort does not mean without effort. Comfort does not merely mean the absence of 'pain' of the sort that tends to come with habitual action or negligence. Find comfort in both feet. Stand so that each foot is evenly in contact with the ground. Stand so that the ankles are not tilting inward or outward to excess. The weight of your body is neither too far forward towards your toes, nor too far back into your heels. Stand so that your face is not held in a frown. Your knees are softly unlocked. Your buttocks are not clenched. The perineum is at ease, as is the space around your bladder. Find an expansiveness around your kidneys and lower belly.

Imagine a pair of shutters on your back, between the shoulders. Let these shutters be wide open, allowing light and space to flood the back body. In the space behind your heart, imagine a pair of windows open inward. On your back, the vast expanse of a mountain range. You're looking out of the open shutters. Behind the heart, a calm, clear antechamber filled with light and lightness. Between your chin and your heart, cocoon something precious. This loving lowering of the face facilitates a lengthening on the back of the neck, allowing energy to rise from the tailbone to the occiput. The skull is light and lifted. The arms are supported magically, as if they are resting on handrails. The shoulders are soft but not slumped. The elbows are unlocked, not bent to excess. The wrists are easy, and the palms are kind. Your jaw and face are ready to smile, but not actually pulling the muscles into a smile. Your eyes are pleased to see whatever is before you. Now, run through this list again, from feet to face. Repeat this until you feel ready to stop, to step away and move on with your day.

There is no expectation of how long you may want to spend in this practice. There is no guideline for progressing from three minutes to fifteen minutes over ten days. Simply try it. Familiarise yourself with this practice of standing, instructing the body to find ease, continually and repeatedly scanning the length of the body, and then move on when you feel ready. The familiarity that comes with frequent practice will reveal to you the benefits that your body needs to draw from this practice. I have no prescriptions for you, but I encourage you to journal your evolving experience of this practice. Stay present to the feedback in your body but do not go searching for any sensations. Let the benefits play out in your life off the mat. Give yourself and your body some time and space to integrate these practices without the need to name or share your experiences.

Qualities of qi and dynamics of movement

Movements used in qigong practices can be broadly categorised into the following spectra:

- expand or shrink

- full or empty

- rise or sink

- accelerate or decelerate

- linear or spiral

- external or internal.

These ideas apply to both the quality of movement and the direction of movement. It is important to remember that these words stem from common parlance in China. While they are obvious and clearly defined terms in English, an exploration of the roots and meanings of these words in Chinese will provide subtler nuances and allow a broader appreciation of what they mean within the native context of qigong practices.

Expand

When we expand, we move through matter and space, we come into contact, we find intimacy. The Chinese character for the verb expand (*kuo*) consists of the component meaning hand, and of another component meaning broad, wide, vast or spread. This second component can also be broken down further into elements meaning a house on a cliff, the contents within it being divided. This demonstrates the capacity of expansion to be external in nature, like the privileged view from a high point, and also to take the form of dividing a single unit into smaller quantities, as when joy is amplified by dividing a cake to share between eight people. An electron microscope can zoom in on a tiny object to a multiple of ten million, while the farthest point sighted in space is some 13 billion light years away. Our attention can expand inwards and outwards like both of these, taking us closer to the object of our focus. By expanding inwards and outwards, we can get close to what is internal and external. As your ribcage expands with a deep breath, visualise the expansion happening at a cellular level throughout your body. See this as a private, personal moment of getting in touch with each little molecule within you. You may also see this as an expansion of the atmosphere of the planet to make deeper contact with your physical body.

Shrink

The Chinese verb to shrink (*suo*) has many facets: to withdraw, to pull back, to recoil, to reduce, to contract, to abbreviate, to compress, to concentrate (a liquid), to tighten and to summarise. As you physically spiral in, or turn your gaze to look within, or curl your fingers into a fist, wrap an arm round, fold forward, bend a leg or curl into a ball on the ground, explore the increased density, strength, tension, weight or concentration that results from the movement. *Suo* is not merely to make something smaller. Be aware of the potential that pools within it for an opposite, expansive movement.

Full

Fullness and satisfaction are synonymous in the Chinese language. The same word is used to mean both that something is crammed to the limit and to be contented, to satisfy and to be satisfied. The simple negative, not full, can be more illustrative, as it means resentful, discontented, dissatisfied. The character *man*, meaning full, is made up of the component for water, the character for ten (the largest digit in Chinese) shown twice and an upturned box, the space within which is occupied. The presence of water is important here. Water always finds a level state. This fullness is one of equanimity and of evenness, of contentment. There is no desire for more. A body of water does not make a hole to indicate its lack. Being full to satisfaction means that there is no more longing, no striving for better, no more feeling that where we are is not enough. Lao Tzu warns us in Chapter 9 of the *Tao Te Ching*:[1]

> Fill your bowl to the brim and it will spill.
> Keep sharpening your knife and it will blunt.

With regular practice, we hone our ability to know when 'enough' becomes 'just right'.

Empty

Through craft, we create tools: bowls, knives, wheels, roofs and bricks, but as described in Chapter 11 of the *Tao Te Ching*, these items gain meaning through their use: 'We work with being, but non-being is what we use.'[2] The empty bowl holds the soup, the knife cuts the meat, the wheel moves the hay, the house allows the family to grow.

Emptiness is not nothing. It is the vacuum that invites life to enter. The word *kong*, meaning empty, also means space, air, sky and fruitless effort. It is made up of components that mean a cave and work. The Chinese character for abyss, which we often think of as an unending void, is depicted as a deep pool with water splashing between two banks. The character used to describe absence or a vacant place is the same character that is used to describe a broken bowl. This character, *que*, is drawn as a hand holding half of a pot. It is an object, but one with no meaningful use. When whole, an empty bowl is useful, but when broken, there is no hope.

The essence of *kong*, of this kind of emptiness, is that it carries the potential for what is possible within its space. So when we try to find

---

1   Mitchell, S. (1988) *Tao Te Ching: A New English Version*. New York: Harper & Row.
2   *Ibid.*

emptiness within a posture, or sometimes just within the space of a limb, the aim is not to disconnect or to make like it is not there. The inverse is what we want to discover: when really free, relaxed, soft, at ease, what can we find possible within the posture?

Rise

The verb to rise in Chinese is also pronounced qi but is written completely differently. *Qi,* meaning to rise, is made up of two components that mean to run and oneself. The word also means to launch, to establish, to set out, to start, to initiate action; and all of these in addition to the most common meaning, which is to get up. Within the component for run are components that mean earth (as in ground), person and a stopping action. This implies a rising from the ground, or the action of pressing against the ground. Simply adding the word for one (*yi*) before *qi* here creates the phrase meaning 'being together in the same place at the same time' (*yi qi*). Presence is implied in the use of the word. Another common use of the word is in the simple apology, *dui bu qi* (which is used to mean 'I am sorry'). *Dui* literally means to face someone or to reply, while *bu* means no, here meaning not able to. Thus, the common phrase meaning simply 'I am sorry' carries, in the way that it is written, a nuance of not being able to rise to the occasion.

When rising within a posture or a movement, therefore, be aware of the integrity and presence that you invite into that moment. Be here, with it, in your body, the moment and the movement.

Sink

The Chinese character for the verb to sink, *chen,* is drawn as water covering a table. It is used to mean to submerge, to immerse, to keep down, to sink, to lower, to drop. It is also used as an adjective to mean deep, profound or heavy. The same character, *chen,* is found in all these phrases: peace (*chen jing*); contemplation or meditation (*chen si*); silence or stillness (*chen ji*); steady, calm and collected (*chen zhuo*); to immerse or soak (*chen jin*); deeply engrossed (*chen mi*); oppressive weather (*chen men*); harsh and critical (*chen zhong*); uncommunicative (*chen mo*). Unmistakable are the implications of a downward trajectory, a weight, a saturation, a concentration, a density, disconnection and solitude. All these examples also indicate there is some *thing* to sink into or be submerged by, be it thought, weather, absence of sound or a topic of obsession. Transformation follows after allowing oneself to be immersed, sunk, saturated. There is a suggestion of treasures to be discovered within the depths.

As you sink into a posture, or dip your hips, or bend your leg, or lower your arm, or find the end of an exhale, observe the density, saturation, stillness and weight of where you are. Observe your reactions to these sensations. Observe the impulse to change, shift or move out of this state.

Accelerate

Kuai ma jia bian is one of many famous four-word Chinese idioms. The four words here are fast, horse, increase and whip. The phrase means to spur on a swift horse. The story stems from a conversation between an old master and his brilliant but lazy student. The master says, 'Imagine you are setting off on a journey with an ox and a horse. Which would you spur on with a whip?' Unhesitating, the student replies, 'The horse, because it is capable of great speed. This is why the horse deserves the encouragement of the whip.' With this metaphor, the student realises his own ability and begins to apply himself.

Two characters are needed to convey the meaning of accelerate: *jia su*, which means add speed. *Su* means velocity or simply fast. *Jia* means add or increase. The same two words also mean expedite, to make something happen faster. Momentum and potential must be present in order to accelerate. The skill we seek is not to speed up merely for the sake of velocity. The skill comes in assessing the capacity for acceleration and the potential to be realised by increasing velocity. This assessment requires wisdom. Maintain awareness of your capacity as you practise, so you can make wise decisions about the speed you are moving at and choose when to capitalise by adding speed and when not to. We will do well to bring the same awareness to any tendency to push, to increase to excess or to stress unnecessarily whilst performing any exercise.

Decelerate

Ning jing zhi yuan is a famous saying by Zhuge Liang, chancellor and regent of the Han state during the Three Kingdoms period (220–280 CE). The phrase means 'enduring accomplishments are achieved by leading a quiet life'. The words literally mean peaceful, stillness (not moving), to deliver, far. This points to the belief that more is accomplished when our actions are not excessive. The Chinese verb to decelerate is written simply by using the two characters meaning reduce and velocity, *jian su*. The important character is *jian*, which is made up of a component meaning ice and the character for salty or miserly. The same word is used in phrases meaning to diet, to depressurise, to delete, to subtract, to lighten, to ease. In qigong we value *ruo*, meaning weakness, or more specifically an absence of resistance. This can be a quality of softness, yielding, surrender, stepping back, vulnerability or humility. While practising, find the opportunity to ease back, to take your foot off the pedal. Explore what may open up and be revealed in the process.

Linear

Unlike yoga asana, the concept of lines in qigong is not about shapes, it is about trajectory. There are seven directions in qigong: northward, southward, eastward, westward, to the centre, upward and downward. Traditionally, we stand in qigong postures with our back towards the north and our face towards the south. This habit has roots in *Feng Shui* and the Five Elements, where the direction of north is associated with the past, our ancestry and the cold winter.

The south is where the future lies. In Chinese, a compass is a dependable needle pointing south, *zhi nan zhen*. During the Han period, Chinese astrology was drafted by observing stars that never set below the horizon (hence, south).

The centre is considered a direction in qigong because it is a point from which we are constantly deviating, and to which we always return. The concept of a contrary movement, a rebound, a return, *fan zhe* in Chinese, is core to qigong. It is the way of nature. As we move in qigong, remember the anchor point of a posture and track where you move relative to this point. There will be a leading point (like your hand, knee or head) and an anchor point (most often your feet). Coming back to centre is like coming home.

There are sharp, quick, directed movements in qigong: a kick, a look, a pointing of a finger, the sweep of an arm, a clear step forward. The linearity here is in the immediacy and singularity of intent. No dawdling, no fuss, no procrastination.

Spiral

Spirals are expressed in our DNA, the nerves of our eyes, a snail shell, the coil of a honeysuckle, the water draining out of a sink, a tropical cyclone, the shape of galaxies. They are also in the structure and movement of the human heart. All mammals and birds have a similar heart structure, where blood is pumped by the two ventricles using a suctioning and ejecting motion. The work of surgeon Dr Francisco Torrent-Guasp shows how the heart's muscle fibres are a single band, the two halves of which spiral into one another to make the two ventricles. As the muscle fibres spiral in opposing directions, so does the pumping action. The blood, therefore, also flows in and out of the heart in movements that coil in and spin out.

There isn't anything to go searching for here, but remember that a spiral movement goes deeper than a twist of the spine, a turn of the head or the roll of a limb. Rolling, spiralling, turning, twisting, the impulse is natural and to be discovered as you move into any shape, and as you stay still. Don't work too hard to find the spiral. Let it reveal itself as you explore and get intimate with your breath and body.

External and internal

The terms *wai dan gong* and *nei dan gong*, referring to complementary and frequently taught practices, may be familiar. *Wai dan* starts by building strength in the limbs on the premise that the energy will then flow from the limbs inward to the centre of the body. The practice of *Wai dan* includes physical movement, massage and acupuncture. *Nei dan* is the inverse, where cultivation of qi starts within the centre of the body on the premise that it will then flow out to the limbs. Its practices include diet, meditation and breathing exercises.

Arguably more important are *wai zhuang* and *nei zhuang*, which are the results, not the styles of training. *Zhuang* is the verb to strengthen. The Chinese character is drawn as split wood and scholar, with these two components indicating robustness beyond physical strengthening. The word is used to describe acts of magnificence, bravery, heroism, glory.

The *jing*, qi and *shen* are governed by the *yi*, our intention. To build strength, we hone our intention. We make skilful choices so that the way in which we use our efforts and energy is not wasteful or hurtful. We stay present in our body and in our lives. We nourish ourselves physically, mentally and emotionally. We keep our body strong and clean. We maintain the body by necessary and available means to enable our organs to thrive and our blood to flow well. This is the ending to the passage from the *Yi Jin Jing* quoted at the start of this book:

> The body which has shape must acquire the shapeless qi, mutually relying and not opposing, in order to generate an indestructible body. If they oppose and do not rely on each other, then the ones with shape will also become without shape.

It takes the combined application of *nei zhuang* and *wai zhuang* to turn strength into bravery, to turn noise into music, to turn food into a family meal, to turn a gesture into an act of devotion. One is meaningless without the other.

Chapter 3

THE QI CIRCULATORY SYSTEM

Part 1: The central meridians

There are two meridians that run along the centre of the body. One extends from the perineum up the front of the torso, and another from the tailbone up the central line of the back and over the skull. Both run down inside the body along the spine. The meridian on the front of the body is called the Conception Vessel, and the one on the back, the Governor Vessel. The Conception Vessel begins at the point on the perineum often called the *moola* or *mula* in yoga practices: the space between the anus and the genitals. The Governor Vessel starts at the tip of the coccyx. The Conception Vessel is regarded as *yin*, feminine; the Governor Vessel as *yang*, masculine. They both have a rising and descending quality as their circuits loop up the surface of the body and down along the spine. If we look at a side-view cross section of the torso, they create a pattern that looks similar to the symbol for infinity, ∞ . These two meridians are deep resources of energy. The energy that resides within the Governor Vessel and Conception Vessel is often used in acupuncture to refresh the flow of qi in the other twelve meridians.

Exercises to stimulate the central meridians

MICROCOSMIC ORBIT BREATH EXERCISE

Preparatory understanding

Before we begin this exercise for the first time, it will be helpful to familiarise ourselves with specific points on the body where we will rest our attention when we move through the practice. The wisdom and correspondences of acupuncture points along these two meridians can provide a cultural context to this practice.

We start in the space of the perineum, between the anus and the genitals. This is the starting point of this practice and, in Chinese medicine, also the starting point of life. This point on the body is called the *Hui Yin*. Here is found a meeting, a coming together (*hui*) of vital essences and life energy (*yin*). It is from the richness of the energy pooled here in the depths of the body that new life is born. This point is the starting point of the Conception Vessel, the feminine energy channel.

The masculine partner to this point on the body sits at the tip of the tailbone or coccyx, where the Governor Vessel begins. This point is called *Chang Qiang*, which carries the image of enduring strength, like that of an arrow that is shot from a bow that has been perfectly and fully drawn. The power harnessed in the drawing of the bow provides the energy for the arrow to fly its fullest distance. The energy that rises from this point is vibrant and vigorous.

Moving up to the sacrum and into the lumbar spine, we find two points of energy that correspond to the creation of life: *Yao Yang Guan* and *Ming Men*. Both of these names carry the character for a gate (*guan*) or a door (*men*), signifying that they are points of exchange, control and release of energy. *Yao Yang Guan* carries the image of a man's desire awakening in his loins. It is, as the name suggests, a vibrant and masculine (*yang*) energy. *Ming Men* corresponds to the energy stored in our kidneys, the essence of life with which we are born. The energy here relates to the drive we have for fully embracing our daily life. It is believed that feeling fully charged in this area of the body, yet also flexible and free, reflects the same qualities in other aspects of our life.

Near where the thoracic spine meets the lumbar is another potent point, called *Zhong Shu*. In English it is translated as Central or Middle

Pivot. *Zhong* is commonly used in Chinese to mean the middle or the centre. The same Chinese character is also used to mean the centre of a target, or a central line dividing two sides. Here, *shu* means pivot, but the word is also used to mean hub. The energy associated with this point is one of coming and going, of ease in the busyness of life, of comfortable flow and willingness to exchange. It seems appropriate that the diaphragm – the muscle that powers the exchange of air in our lungs – connects to the spine just under this point.

Behind the heart-centre are the points *Ling Tai* and *Shen Dao*. To understand the energy of these points, imagine you are standing on the roof of a tower. From here you see gardens, and then fields, beyond which lie forests, all full of life. There has been recent rainfall. You can smell the freshness and vitality in the air and on your skin. You can see it on the plants and hear the animals frolicking in the freshness. From where you are standing you can see the horizon in every direction. The sky is uninterrupted; the view is clear. From the tower you see your path ahead, leading through the garden, fields and forest into the distance. The path is clear and sure; there are no byways or tracks that may steer you off course. You feel certain and secure in the knowledge that you are in the right place.

As we ascend further up the spine, a significant point of transition is at the base of the cervical spine. This point is called *Da Zhui* or Great Hammer. This is a point used in acupuncture to awaken and enliven *yang* energy in the body. As we move upwards, from the torso – the region of earthly concerns – into the head – the region of heavenly or spiritual pursuits – this is an important transition point. *Da* is the word for big, but it also means a person with maturity and wisdom. *Zhui* means vertebrae first, but also means to strike, a mallet or a hammer. It carries an image of solidity and strength. This point, given its location, is associated with life and death. Whether in the breaking of a person's neck or the finality of a judge's gavel, the energy here is one of urgency, vitality. It suggests a mature awareness of the great importance of what happens next on the journey of life.

Three points on the head capture the spirit carried by this meridian as it rises over the skull: *Feng Fu* (Wind Palace), *Bai Hui* (One Hundred Meetings) and *Yin Tang* (Hall of Impressions). *Feng Fu* is at the occiput, where the neck meets the base of the skull. This point corresponds to clarity and potency, like a very clean, well-organised, fully stocked warehouse. *Bai Hui* is located on the centre line of the skull (sagittal suture), slightly behind the crest of the skull (coronal suture). *Hui* means a meeting. Here is the coming together of the bones of the skull, signifying unity and singular strength. *Yin* in *Yin Tang* means to imprint, to make a clear impression. It also means a seal or a stamp. It is located right between the eyebrows, where blessings are often placed on one's forehead. It corresponds to the third eye in some traditions, and is sometimes called the upper *dantian* (upper font of energy) in qigong. In acupuncture this point is used to dissolve mental chaos and to decongest the sinus area. This gives us an insight into the energy found at *Yin Tang*: spaciousness, calm, clarity of purpose and identity.

Moving down into the mouth and throat, we come to points on the Conception Vessel. The names of some of the points in the mouth and throat clearly indicate the corresponding energy: *Cheng Jiang* (Receiving of Broth), *Lian Quan* (Angled Spring) and *Tian Tu* (Heaven Rushes Out). This is an area bursting with vital, nourishing, essential fluid. This refers to the fluency and ease of speech, as well as to that which we take into our lives.

In the space from the base of the sternum to the upper edge of the pectoral muscles are energy points that correspond to the heart. The energy here is the energy of great harmony, of warm sunlight, of respect, of propriety and of wisdom. The names of these points all carry an indication of a courtyard, a palace or a hall, to reflect the importance of a protected space where the heart can reside and from which it can rule. We are also reminded of the luxurious trappings of sovereignty by these names: *Yu Tang* (Jade Court), *Zi Gong* (Purple Palace) and *Xuan Ji* (Jade and Irregular Pearl). In this space, we are invited to discern and hold what is of value in our heart.

Between the sternum and the navel are points corresponding to the energy required for processing, movement and storage. The names of these points have characters for gateways (*que*), ducts and cavities (*wan*): *Shen Que, Ju Que, Shang Wan, Zhong Wan, Xia Wan*. This area of the body is where our food and thoughts are processed, transformed into usable energy and then channelled or stored as needed. A healthy expression of the energy here would be one of true cooperation, of great freedom and ease amid the busyness.

Coming into the lower belly, we arrive at a region of deep, abundant reserves. This region is paralleled by the great abundance contained in the oceans of the world – so vast and deep that much remains unknown and undiscovered. These reserves are regulated by a series of gates and doorways: *Shi Men* (Stone Gateway) and *Guan Yuan* (First or Original Mountain Pass). We are once again in the presence of vital essences, of energy that contains the potential for creating new life. Many of the mysteries of life on land are unlocked through learning about life in the deepest ocean. Likewise, the shape of our lives starts with what is deep within our bones. This ancestral inheritance is reflected in the limitations and strengths that we carry through our lives. The qualities corresponding to this space are reverence, drive, commitment, strength of will and respect for our ability to access these reserves. Bring your awareness of these qualities into the flesh, the bones and the fluids in your lower belly.

You may want to give yourself time to further explore these meridians and the energy points on them. Perhaps, choose one quality corresponding to each of these areas as you now begin to practise this Microcosmic Orbit exercise.

The exercise

Sit or stand comfortably. Find your feet and make any adjustments that you need to feel comfortable. Be sufficiently comfortable to sustain this position for the duration of the practice, which could be three to five minutes as you start to learn it. Over time, this can extend to ten or fifteen minutes.

Visualise the central line of your body. If possible, maybe even feel the volume of the spine up and down the centre of your torso. Become aware of the volume of space within the torso. The space in your throat, in your chest, all the way around your ribcage. Feel the density of your internal organs: your stomach, your liver, the intestines, the kidneys. Tune in to your breathing. Breathe normally as you begin this practice, allowing the lungs, belly and chest to move without pressure or expectation. Explore the space of your throat, your mouth and your face. Go deeper into the cavities of your face: your eye sockets, your sinuses, your ears, the space in your skull. Build your sensitivity to the space within your body from the top of the head down to the perineum. If you are coming to this practice for the first time, this exploration itself can already be a deep and powerful exercise that can take three to five minutes. If you feel the need to stop at this point, please stop. Practise this body scan regularly, until tuning in to this inner space becomes comfortable, effortless and frictionless for you. Once this becomes familiar, you can progress to the next phase of this exercise.

In this next phase of the practice, we trace a line up the back of the spine, starting from the tailbone, up and over the top of the head, down the front of the body and through the heart, before descending to arrive at the perineum. We pause along the way at the points described above for a few breaths or more. At each point, as we pause we bring our awareness to its corresponding qualities. There is a lot to take in, and it may not be possible to remember all the qualities at once. I encourage you to distil the descriptions provided above into a few words that resonate for you. This way, you will have a simpler set of words to focus on during the meditation. I often teach this with only four points of focus: tailbone, head, heart and lower belly. Remember, the circuit starts in the tailbone, you rise up the back of the spine, over the head, down to the heart and then end by anchoring yourself back in the belly. If for any reason you should feel light-headed whilst practising this, only practise the downward part of the circuit, from the top of the head down to the lower belly.

MACROCOSMIC ORBIT 1

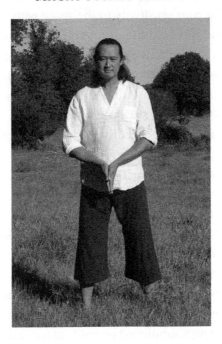

This is a movement from the *Shibashi* (second sequence).

Stand in Horse Stance. The palms are touching – fully touching – at the level of the lower belly, with the fingers pointing down to the earth. The movement of the hands will trace a circuit upwards, outwards and then downwards along the central axis of the torso. To start, keep your fingers pointing down as you raise your hands towards the base of the sternum. The fingers will start to point forward. Continue to raise the hands a little more, up to the heart-centre. Then send the hands and arms forward, with the fingers leading. Finally, bring the hands back down to the lower belly. Keep the palms fully touching throughout the movement, tracing this somewhat circular shape in alignment with the central axis of your torso. Keep your shoulders and elbows relaxed and soft as you move your arms. You can harmonise your breathing with the circular movement of the hands, using one full breath cycle for one circuit. I find it most comfortable to inhale on the way up and exhale as the arms move forward and down. If your breath is shallow, unhook the breath cycle from the movement. Keep the movement present, slow and constant, but breathe freely and easily.

For a more challenging variation of this exercise, sit deeper in Horse

Stance. Keep your knees aligned over your feet, angled outwards at about 45°. If you are building up to a long hold here, try pumping the legs on each cycle: rise out of the Deep Horse Stance on inhale and sink back down on exhale. After a few rounds like this, you can maintain the legs in the deeper position while the arms continue for a few more cycles. Remember to keep the shoulders and elbows relaxed throughout.

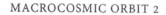

MACROCOSMIC ORBIT 2

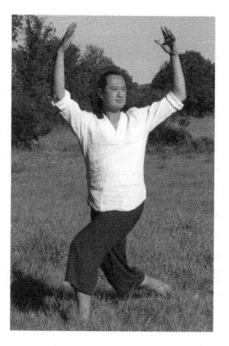

The image above shows the movement of the torso and arms while in a lunge.

Stand evenly. We start by establishing the movement for the arms.

On inhale, raise the arms out to the sides and up to the sky, allowing the palms to face one another as they arrive. On exhale, we bring the hands down in front of the torso, along the central line of the body. As the hands come down, both palms face the body but one is aligned behind the other, so that one hand is closer to the body and the other is a few inches in front of it. It doesn't matter which hand is nearer the body – do what feels instinctively right for you. Do this a few times to establish the movement.

When you feel ready to move on, as you raise your arms on inhale, turn the chest to the right. This means that your left arm will now be reaching forward, and the right arm is reaching behind you. Keep your feet anchored, pointing forward. On exhale, bring the chest back to centre, facing forward, and lower the hands along the central axis of the body. Repeat on the other side.

The movement of the hands mimics the trajectory of the Governor and Conception Vessels – one in front and one behind – as they travel up and down the central axis of the torso. As you move the arms, stay present to the space outside the torso and the space within it. Notice how you are moving in the space around you and within your torso. Your feet stay deeply rooted, the crown of your head – around the point of the *Bai Hui* – is aligned to the sky. Stay present to how you are being held between earth and sky as you navigate the space in front, behind and on either side of you. Visualise the loop of the circuits as you move and breathe. Especially when the hands are moving down through the centre, imagine them lightly brushing the spine deep within you.

The two Macrocosmic Orbit exercises can be performed with the legs in a deep lunge, in Chair Pose or in Temple Pose. For a more dynamic movement, you can pump the legs while you circle the arms. These exercises can be incorporated into sequences that emphasise spinal extension, flexion and rotation.

Part 2: The Emperor and his Ministers

There are twelve other meridians that link throughout the body and that correspond to specific organ systems and functions. There is a hierarchy: the Heart is the 'Emperor', and the other 11 meridians each serve the Emperor in equal measure. All these twelve meridians have sections called 'superficial channels', meaning that they are near the surface of the skin, and 'deep channels', meaning that they are not reachable with an acupuncture needle because they are too deep in the body. When a meridian is being discussed in this book, it will be the superficial channel that is being referenced unless the converse is stated. Although each meridian will be described in the singular, all twelve meridians are bilateral at the superficial level, meaning that they run on both the left and right sides of the body.

You can imagine these meridians as electricity cables and water pipes that run throughout a house. The qi is the electric current and the water. If there is a faulty connection or a blockage along the way, qi doesn't flow through. This blockage shows up as illness or dis-ease. The body functions best when all channels are fully connected and when energy flows freely and evenly. When there is an excess or a deficit of energy in any channel, symptoms will appear. These symptoms may be physical, mental or emotional. Life is how we use the energy that flows through us, so a disturbance in energy flow can consequently show up as a disturbance in any aspect of our life.

The twelve meridians connect to each other on the superficial level. At the deeper level, they connect to their corresponding organs. There is a sequence to these twelve meridians in the way that they connect and a direction of flow for each of them. When we observe how these lines feed into each other and traverse the body, we understand better how to sequence movements and postures accordingly.

We start at the Heart, the 'Emperor'. The Heart is simple and singular in function. It is direct and humble. These qualities are reflected in the path of the Heart meridian. This meridian starts at the armpit where the pectoralis major overlaps the heads of the bicep muscles. The meridian flows down the inner seam of the arm to the little finger where it meets the Small Intestine meridian. There are only nine acupuncture points on the Heart meridian. The Heart in Chinese medicine is seen as the supreme controller of body, mind and spirit. Its role is to establish order and to command. All the other meridians serve the Heart, and the Heart, in return, works hard to preserve and protect all the other meridians on which it relies. The Heart must be preserved at all costs, or else life ends. If the Heart is in good health, all other problems are manageable.

The Small Intestine meridian starts at the outer edge of the little finger, runs along the seam of the hand to the wrist and continues up the outside of the arm into the back of the upper arm. From there it rises into the crease of the armpit on the back of the body and then zigzags along the scapula before climbing up the side of the neck to the cheek. Finally, it turns back to end at the ear. The role of the Small Intestine is to separate the pure from the impure. It extracts the pure qi from what is ingested by the body and sends what is left down to the colon. This does not only apply to food; the Small Intestine sifts through everything we take in via our senses and our thoughts, recognises what is worth keeping and discards the pollutants.

The Small Intestine meridian connects to the Bladder meridian, which starts deep in the eye socket on the side of the nose. The Bladder meridian is the longest meridian on the body and has 67 acupuncture points. It runs the entire length of the body, from the eyes, over the scalp, down the back of the torso, into the buttocks and down the back of the legs and ends in the little toe. This meridian covers more ground than any of the others because it also splits into parallel lines several times on its journey from head to toe. The section of the Bladder meridian on the back of the torso has spurs connecting to all the other meridians. The role of the Bladder meridian is to control the storage and elimination of water, as fluid is what makes up the greater part of the body.

The Bladder meridian ends in the little toe, and the Kidney meridian starts in the sole of the foot. *Yong Quan* (Bubbling Spring) is an important point for establishing our connection to the earth in the standing postures of qigong. This point is between the second and third metatarsal bones, about a third of the way down from the toes on the sole of the foot. You'll find it easily if you massage the sole of your foot. Under the ball of the foot, there is usually a soft dip: this is *Yong Quan*. The meridian rises to the inner arch of the foot under the navicular bone and then up and around the ankle bone. It continues rising along the inner leg into the groin. The kidneys hold the intelligence and control of life's essential juices. The qi we inherit from the DNA of the sperm and egg is stored in the kidneys and is regulated by this meridian. The meridian continues up the trunk through the reproductive organs, connecting to the Conception Vessel in the lower belly and the Governor Vessel on the lumbar spine. The Kidney meridian continues up the front of the torso under the diaphragm and goes all the way up into the clavicles.

On the chest, the Kidney meridian sends a spur to connect with the Pericardium meridian. The pericardium is a fibrous layer that wraps the heart and heart vessels. In Chinese medicine, it functions as the heart protector, absorbing any physical and emotional shocks to the heart. It is, in fact, often called the Heart Protector meridian. The Pericardium meridian starts beside the nipple, rises to the armpit and continues down the arm between the bicep muscles, between the radial tendons, all the way to the centre of the palm and into the middle finger. The point in the middle of the palm, *Lao Gong* (Palace of Toil), is used as an alignment point in qigong. It is a major energy point that corresponds to the Fire element. This point represents a 'palace' where the *shen* or spirit can reside and refresh itself. This meridian also regulates our relationship with sex, sexuality and sexual propriety: note the sensitivity and intimacy experienced in touching the inner arm and the centre of our palms. A useful practice in qigong is to observe how you use your hands, how you touch things as you go about daily life and even how you touch the people in your life. Many students feel heat in their palms when practising qigong. Building awareness and sensitivity in your hands will greatly increase your overall sensitivity to sensations of energy in qigong practice.

Here we are reminded of the benefits of cultivating a qigong practice. It harnesses energy for us to use in our lives. It is not like a big savings account, where we want to bank every penny we can for a rainy day. A daily qigong practice will provide a steady, easy flow of cash for spending readily on all our activity, with neither fear of depletion nor risk of excess.

The Triple Heater is the counterpart to the Pericardium. The Triple Heater does not have a physical manifestation in the form of organ tissue or structure but is a function and indicator of the working of the three centres of heat in the body. The three centres of heat are in the lower belly, the solar plexus and the chest. Nourishment is received in the stomach, which is located in the solar plexus region. Heat is provided from the lower belly, where the kidneys are located. The vapours from the cooking process rise to the chest, the region of the lungs and heart, where they are used and distributed. When the Triple Heater is functioning well, these three spaces work efficiently. Energy and heat are distributed evenly throughout the body. The entire being can relax, and life is joyous. The meridian starts beside the nail bed on the outer edge of the ring finger. It rises along the outside of the arm, up the shoulder and on to the neck. It circles behind the ear up to the outer edge of the eye socket.

The Gallbladder meridian picks up the baton from the Triple Heater at the edge of the eye socket, zigzags over the scalp to the base of the skull, comes forward over the shoulder to the side of the ribs, zigzags down to the buttocks and then flows down the outer seam of the leg and into the fourth toe. In total, 20 out of 44 acupuncture points on this meridian are located on the head. This may indicate the influence of the Gallbladder on our ability to make wise judgements and swift, clear decisions. In English and in Chinese, the phrase 'to have the gall' is used to indicate the audacity of a certain decision or action. When we say that something is 'galling', it usually means that the situation is incredibly vexing or provocative. Both these examples indicate the anticipation of a suitable response, without which inequity would persist. With a healthily functioning Gallbladder meridian, we are freely and readily able to respond to any situation with fair judgements and take honourable actions. The names of the following points capture the spirit of this meridian well: *Tian Chong* (With the Full Force of Heaven), *Wei Dao* (Binding Path), *Zheng Ying* (Correct Way of Being), *Ri Yue* (Sun and Moon), *Guang Ming* (Bright and Clear), *Yang Ling Quan* (Spring of Yang Energy) and *Qiu Xu* (A Mound in the Wilderness).

The Liver meridian picks up the line. Starting on the lateral edge of the big toenail, this meridian rises between the first and second metatarsal bones into the ankle and then continues up the inside of the leg along the medial edge of the tibia and the femur. Like the Kidney meridian, it moves deep in the thigh up into the groin, over the inguinal crease and then zigzags under the side ribs into the diaphragm. The channel continues deep in the body up to the eye. The Liver meridian is responsible for our ability to have a vision, make a plan and put it into action. It is associated with our ability to stand up and step forward. This is implied by the name of the first and last points on the meridian: *Da Dun* (Great Esteem) and *Qi Men* (Gate of Hope). *Da Dun* is often used to treat virility and fertility issues in men. *Qi Men* is a point used to encourage a stronger connection with the in-breath and to promote flow of qi up into the lungs.

The Lung meridian is next, starting near the top of the lungs on the upper edge of the pectoral muscle. It rises into the dip under the clavicle, goes over the front of the shoulder and continues along the radial side of the arm to the thumb. The Lung meridian is responsible for receiving the pure qi from the heavens. More importantly, it is responsible for the literal and metaphorical inspiration in our body and in our life. It governs our ability to transcend the mundane. The Lung provides the spark that enables us to identify, obtain and appreciate virtue and excellence in spirit and in kind. The names of a few points on the clavicle and shoulder indicate the Lung meridian's role in helping us stay connected to the divine: *Yun Men* (Gateway of Clouds), *Tian Fu* (Celestial Palace) and *Xia Bai* (Valiant White).

The Large Intestine meridian starts in the tip of the index finger and runs up along the seam of the forearm into the elbow crease. It then continues up into the shoulder and neck, and terminates beside the nostril. A key point on this meridian is *He Gu* (A Union of Valleys), located where the index finger and thumb meet. The location of the point and its name indicate a strong holding power. This point is often known as the ultimate 'letting-go' point. The primary function of the Large Intestine meridian is to decide what to let go of and what to retain, such as trace minerals. Anything that is not of value is encouraged to pass through. Imagine spotting a diamond lying in the sand: you pick it up in your fingers, you let all the grains of sand fall away and you are left holding your prize. Much more meaningful than simply 'letting go', this meridian teaches us to identify and treasure what is of greatest value and benefit, and to direct our energy into retaining these things. Everything else falls away naturally.

The Large Intestine meridian links to the Stomach meridian, which begins under the eye socket. The Stomach meridian travels down to the corners of the mouth, up the side of the head above the ears and then down to the throat. This section of the meridian is particularly important, as it indicates the kind of nourishment that the Stomach is responsible for processing: everything we take in through our eyes, through our mouth and through our mind. The meridian continues down the nipple line on the torso, straight down the front of the legs and through the middle of the foot and ends in the second toe. The shape of the meridian indicates that a clear passage is necessary for the healthy functioning of this meridian. Indigestion, be it physical or mental churn, is an expression of the Stomach not being able to pass through what has been taken in. This may be caused by taking in too much, by insufficient lubrication or by obsessiveness and control issues. For nourishment to be useful, it must be digested and passed through to the Spleen.

The Spleen meridian is responsible for the distribution of qi. Whatever the Spleen receives from the Stomach is transformed into usable energy and distributed throughout the body via the blood. Poor health in the Spleen may present as blood clots, blood disorders, fibroids or haemorrhoids. *Xue Hai* (Sea of Blood) is a point located on the thigh above the knee that is often used by acupuncturists to address issues such as dysmenorrhea and amenorrhea. The Spleen meridian starts in the medial edge of the big toe and sweeps up the inside of the leg, where it shares the line with the Liver meridian up into the torso. The meridian continues up the outer seam of the torso to the armpit and then drops down into the side ribs at the level of the heart, where it connects to the start of the Heart meridian. This completes the circuit of the twelve meridians.

Enjoy nurturing your awareness of this circuit and the trajectory of these meridian lines, remembering the following:

- These twelve meridians form one continuous loop.

- The effects of activating or stimulating any one meridian will ripple through to the others.

- Joining points are areas where blockages can happen. Acupuncture and Chinese medicine have specific protocols to address these blockages.

- In the context of qigong and yoga, knowing where meridians join one another provides an excellent framework for creating sequences to strengthen weak points or to free up blockages.

Chapter 4

EXERCISES TO STIMULATE THE MERIDIANS

Heart meridian

The function of the Heart is to be the supreme ruler of life.

Separating Clouds

This movement stimulates the superficial and deep channels of the Heart meridian.

Stand evenly and position your hands one over the other, a few inches in front of your heart-centre. Align the very centre of your palms – the *Lao Gong* point – maintaining a gap of a couple of inches between each hand. Before moving, pause here for a moment, allowing your attention to settle in the space of your heart and in your hands.

To start the movement, lower your hands to the level of the lower belly. On inhale, reach both arms forward with your palms facing up and then curl your fingers inwards towards your heart, leading with the little finger. Bring your hands towards your heart in a gathering gesture, as if to say, 'Come on over!' On exhale, let both hands descend along the central line of your body. The backs of your hands look at each other as they move down from your heart to your lower belly.

On the next inhale, send your arms outwards to the sides, up to the level of your shoulders, with the palms facing down. On exhale, return your hands to your lower belly. Start the cycle again from here. Observe the meridian line, which runs from the front of your armpits to the little fingers as you move your arms. Repeat the sequence for three to five minutes. When done, bring the hands back to your heart-centre, keeping the *Lao Gong* points aligned.

The circular arm movements in this exercise mirror the flow of blood through the heart muscle: receiving and sending out what comes up and into the heart. It is a simple, rhythmic movement, which when aligned with the breath, can become meditative, soothing and refreshing. You may find that once you establish the momentum of this exercise, the end of one cycle flows seamlessly into the next.

This is an excellent exercise to use as a precursor to Sun Salutations. I often practise with a mantra that has two parts. For example, as I bring my hands in towards my heart, I say to myself, 'Now, all is well.' As I bring my arms out to the sides, I say, 'May all beings be well.'

Golden Rooster Shakes His Wings

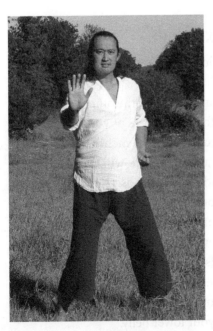 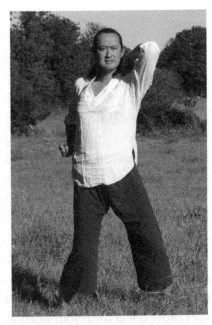

Start in Horse Stance with your hands in front of your chest, the left hand in front of the right and the palms facing the heart and aligning the *Lao Gong* points. The hands are floating in front of the chest, not touching the body. Rotate the left hand and press the left palm forward, as though you want to stop someone. At the same time, bring your right elbow down beside you and pull it back. Your right hand is at the level of the waist.

Now, swing your right elbow forward and up, keeping it bent. As you do this, pull your left elbow back and down, bringing your hand to the waist and keeping the palm open. On exhale, bring both hands back to the heart-centre, this time with the right hand in front of the left. Stay here for the inhale. On exhale, press the right palm forward as you pull the left arm back. On inhale, swing the left elbow forward and up. Bring your right elbow back down at the same time. On exhale, return to centre. Continue this exercise, alternating the arms each time. Stay present to any sensations along the Heart meridian, along the inner seam of the arm from the armpit to the little finger. Observe any warmth or heat building in your chest and your hands. As you stimulate the meridians, you may experience slight tingling in your hands or fingers, sometimes along the meridian line. If you experience any pain or shortness of breath during this or any exercise, stop and rest.

In this exercise, breath quality is key. The first exhale is short and sharp. Use a strong exhale as you press one palm out and pull the other arm in. The inhale as you swing your elbow up is similarly sharp and quick. You may want to try holding this inhale a moment longer, before letting the breath out slowly and fully as the hands come back down. Try sequencing this exercise into classes with twists and arm balances to stimulate heat and vigour.

Sparrowhawk Takes Flight

The full form of this exercise is executed while standing on one leg. As you begin exploring this movement, keep to standing on both legs until you become familiar with how the arms and chest move. Once the upper body movements take less effort, try the exercise while standing on one leg. I will indicate in the instructions below how and when to move from one leg to the other.

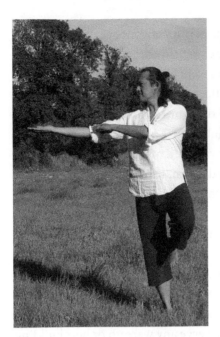 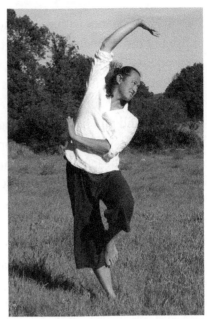

Start in a comfortable Horse Stance. Don't take the feet too far apart, but allow space between the legs so that both feet feel equally and fully in contact with the ground. The palms are held one in front of the other facing the heart-centre, aligned at the *Lao Gong*. On inhale, swing the right arm forward and out to the side, with the palm open, as you would if you were offering a gift to someone standing beside you. Bring the left hand to rest lightly on the inner crease of the right elbow.

On exhale, circle the right arm overhead, turning the torso to look left. The weight of the body will naturally shift into the right leg. As you make this gesture, press both palms away from the body: the right palm overhead towards the sky; the left palm facing to the right and leading your left arm across your chest. Both hands are folded back at the wrist.

On inhale, move your weight back to centre, the torso facing forwards, and bring the left hand in front of the belly with the palm looking upward. Turn the right palm (still above the head) to face down, so that the palms are looking at one another. On exhale, bring the hands back to the heart-centre, aligning the palms at *Lao Gong*.

Now, repeat the movement to the other side. On inhale, swing the left arm out, palm open, offering a precious gift. The right hand comes to rest lightly on the inner crease of the left elbow. On exhale, circle the left arm overhead, turning the chest to look to the right. Press both palms away from the body: left palm to the sky; right palm pressing past your chest to the left. On inhale, turn back to centre, left hand above, right hand at the belly. Turn the palms to face one another. On exhale, bring the hands back to the heart. Repeat the movement until it becomes familiar. Notice whether there is any bias towards one side, or whether your body feels equally comfortable performing this exercise on both sides. When these movements in the upper body become smooth and effortless, you can introduce the leg movements, which are as follows.

When you extend your right arm out to the side, place your body weight on your right leg. Raise your left knee forward so that the inside of the left foot rests on the inner edge of the right leg, either alongside the calf or beside the knee. If balance is challenging for you, try placing your left heel just above the right ankle. Try not to tense your legs. Stay on one leg as you swing your arm overhead. When you eventually bring your hands back down to the heart-centre, lower the lifted leg and relax evenly onto both legs. It is important to stay stable as you move. Having your leg higher up does not mean you are any better at this exercise. Avoid any temptation to overreach. Stay open to the flow of energy and, with time and practice, let your body show you what it is capable of.

For advanced students, this exercise can be used as a transition pose, whether in and out of Sun Salutations, or from Warrior poses to standing balances.

Small Intestine meridian

*The function of the Small Intestine is to
separate the pure from the impure.*

Small Intestine Exercise 1

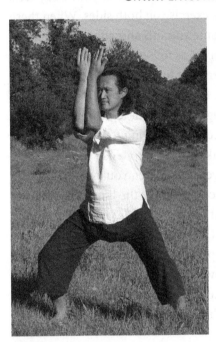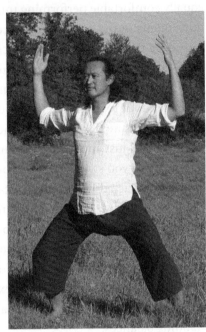

Stand in Horse Stance. Bend your arms so your forearms are in front of your face, with the fingers pointing up. Your elbows are at the level of your armpits. Turn your forearms so you can see your palms. The little fingers can touch along the seam of your hand. Perhaps take a moment to visualise the trajectory of the meridian from the tip of the little finger up the arms, over the shoulders, up the neck into the ear. On inhale, separate the forearms and open your chest. Keep your arms bent, and keep your elbows at the same level. Turn your head to look to the side. On exhale, bring the forearms back together. Turn to face forward. On inhale, open the arms again, and turn to look the other way. On exhale, come back to centre. If it feels possible for you, when you open your arms, lightly squeeze the shoulder blades towards each other on your back. Do not do this if it causes any pain. This exercise can be performed in Deep Horse Stance for a stronger variation.

This exercise can also be used as variations to standing postures such as Pyramid Pose, Warrior 1 and Tree Pose, or seated in Hero's Pose.

Small Intestine Exercise 2

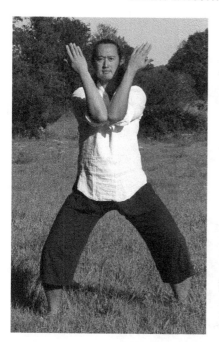 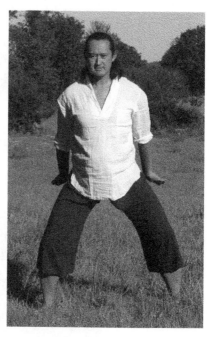

Stand comfortably and evenly in Horse Stance. Bring your forearms to the level of your face, with your fingers pointing up and your palms towards your face. Your elbows are at the level of your armpits. Let your elbows lightly touch, but take your hands away from each other, forming a 'V' shape with the forearms.

On exhale, slowly bring your forearms together, as if zipping them up from the elbows to the tips of the little fingers. As the little fingers touch, the elbows separate. Lower your arms and reach down and back behind you. Turn the palms out so that the backs of your hands look at each other.

On inhale, roll your arms out to the sides to bring them forward. Bring the elbows to touch once again at the level of your armpits. Repeat the cycle, continuing to move your arms slowly in this circular motion. If it does not feel comfortable to align the movement with your breath, breathe naturally and freely, but keep the pace of movement slow and steady.

When performing this exercise seated, prop the sitting bones up on a bolster or some bricks so that the pelvic bowl can freely rock forwards and back with each cycle.

Swimming Dragon variation

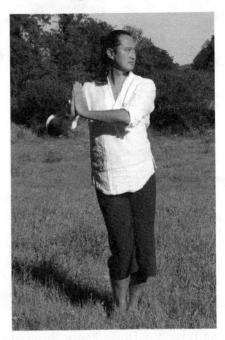

Bring your palms to touch in front of your heart-centre, fingers pointing upward. If possible, stand with your feet together. Gaze softly forward. Find your breath. On exhale, turn your head to the right. At the same time, move your hands to the left and towards the left armpit. Keep the palms touching and keep your hands at the same level. On inhale, bring your gaze and your hands back to the centre. On exhale, turn your head to the left and move your hands over to the right. On inhale, return to centre. You can keep the hands the same distance in front of the body throughout, or have them further away from the chest at the centre so that their movement makes an arc from one armpit to the other.

If it feels comfortable for your shoulders, move continuously from side to side, sweeping your arms forward in an arc. Find a rhythm for your breath that feels sustainable. Once this movement is established and feels comfortable, you can introduce this further movement in the torso and legs: on exhale, as you turn your head, let your chest follow in the same direction. This deepens the rotation and stretch between the hands and the direction you are turning towards. Bend the knees lightly and sink your hips. On inhale, bring yourself back to centre. Repeat evenly on both sides.

This exercise is a useful warm up for twists or as a transition in and out of poses such as Eagle Pose, Chair Pose, Flying Pigeon Pose and Side Crow Pose.

Bladder meridian

The function of the Bladder is to control the flow and storage of water.

The Bladder meridian is closely linked to the nervous system. It supports every meridian by providing direct pathways to fluid for each of them. As a result, it has wide-reaching influence. If you look at a diagram of the meridian, you will see how it runs concurrently with the nervous system. The Bladder meridian corresponds to our instinct to flee, fight or freeze in the presence of danger. The best way to bring qi to the Bladder meridian is by resting. Practices such as Yoga Nidra, Restorative Yoga and Yin Yoga are excellent ways to refresh the flow of qi in the Bladder meridian. There are schools of qigong that, as in yoga, teach *Fang Song Gong*, meaning the qigong of relaxation, as a discipline in its own right.

The Chinese use the words *fang song* to mean relax. The word *fang* means to release, and *song* means to loosen. This approach to relaxation is a conscious retreat from any emotional or muscular tightening. It is practised as a skill, even in the absence of any great tension. This is not about ignoring or forgetting the causes of stress for a period of time, neither is it about occupying the mind with a distraction. The skill is to choose actively to stay loose and free. With practice, this state becomes easily accessible when we find ourselves face to face with tension.

Becoming fluent in frequent and comfortable rest is not something that most of us have ever considered to be a necessary life skill. However, if we look at global statistics on depression, the use of sleep medication and incidences of domestic violence, road rage, relationship breakdown and suicide, it would seem that human beings would benefit greatly from learning to relax more easily.

Whether by lying down, sitting or standing, conscious resting is an excellent way to recharge the flow of energy through the Bladder meridian and calm the nervous system. The following yoga postures are effective tools for rebalancing qi in the Bladder meridian:

- Standing or Seated Forward Fold

- Pyramid Pose

- Standing or Seated Wide-Legged Forward Fold

- Legs Up The Wall

- Happy Baby Pose

- Supported Shoulderstand (with sufficient warm up)

- Plough Pose (with sufficient warm up)

- Child's Pose

- Corpse Pose

- Downward-Facing Corpse Pose.

Alongside all these, there are ways to calm the nervous system and promote flow in the Bladder meridian using movement. Here is a sequence for an advanced flowing yoga class:

1. Start in Standing Forward Fold.

2. Bend your knees deeply and roll back. Rock forward into a squat, and lift your hips into Standing Forward Fold. Repeat this a few times to build momentum, then at an appropriate moment, roll back with enough momentum to lift your legs and hips into Supported Shoulderstand.

3. Repeat this several times, rolling forward into Standing Forward Fold, and back into Supported Shoulderstand.

4. Progress from Supported Shoulderstand into Plough Pose.

5. Finally, roll onto the back for Happy Baby Pose.

This should *not* be attempted by anyone with any neck, shoulder or spinal disc injuries, or anyone with conditions aggravated by deep forward folds and inversions.

Kidney meridian

*The function of the Kidneys is to store
and dispense the essence of life.*

Exercises from Wild Goose qigong

These exercises are from the Wild Goose tradition, a series of movements originating in the Kunlun mountains. The following exercises have been extracted from the first set of 64 movements to create a mini sequence specifically for stimulating the kidneys. This is a useful warm up for classes that focus on forward folds.

WILD GOOSE: OPENING WINGS, FOLDING NEST, SHAKING WINGS

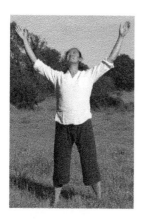 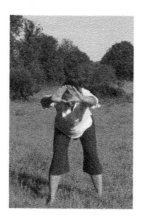 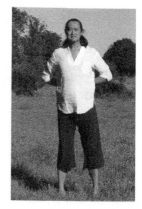

Stand evenly. Reach your arms forward and up, opening them into a 'V' as you reach to the sky. Lean back slightly and pause for a breath. Be careful not to strain your back. Bring the arms forward and bring the palms to your belly, with the thumbs and index fingers touching to form a diamond. Stay here for a breath. Next, keeping the hands in a diamond shape, turn the palms forward and press the hands forward, folding forward at the hips as you extend your arms. Keep your legs steady. Stay here for a breath.

On inhale, stand back up and sweep your arms out, bringing the backs of your hands to your kidneys. At the same time, lift your heels. As you drop your heels on an exhale, brush the backs of your hands (fingertips pointing to your armpits) past your sides to bring them forward to a natural hanging position. Repeat this sequence three or four times and then move on to the next exercise.

WILD GOOSE: CROSS WINGS TO TOUCH THE GROUND

Interlace your fingers and bring the palms of your hands up to your chest. Fold forward from the hips, pressing your palms down to the ground between your feet. Come half way up, bringing the hands to the chest and then press down towards the left foot. Come half way up and press down again between your feet. Come half way up and press down towards the right foot. Once again, come half way up and press down between your feet. Stand back up and release your hands.

WILD GOOSE: FLY OVER WATER

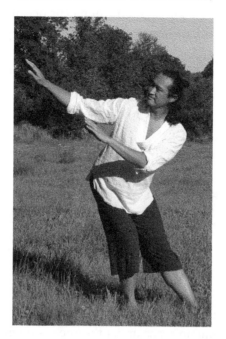

Step your left foot forward, keep your weight on the right leg and bend your right knee slightly. Extend both arms to the right and then sweep them in an arc down towards the ground, hinging forward at the hips and then up to the left. Take a step forward with your right foot. Keep your weight in the left leg and bend the knee lightly. Sweep the arms down in an arc from the left to the right, once again hinging forward at the hips. Repeat seven times, taking a step forward each time.

WILD GOOSE: PLACE WINGS ON BACK

Standing evenly, place the backs of your hands on your lower back, at the level of your kidneys. Lightly rub your lower back, alternating between circular and vertical gestures with the backs of your hands. This movement stimulates four points located here on the lower back that correspond to the health and vitality of the kidneys: *Shen Shu, Qi Hai Shu, Huang Men* and *Zhi Shi*.

Shen here refers to the kidneys. The kidneys store the vital energy inherited from our ancestors. *Shu* means a transfer, an exchange or a liaison. This point on the lower back is a point of direct access to the resources stored in the kidneys. *Qi Hai* means ocean or sea of qi. This point is a link to the Conception Vessel and the energy used for manifesting life. *Huang Men* is a doorway to vitality linked with the function of the diaphragm, the muscle that enables the exchange of gases through each breath. *Zhi* means aspiration, ambition, ideal or will. The character is drawn to indicate growth that stems from the heart. *Shi* is a room in a home. The imagery of this point is reminiscent of the dreams and ambitions of a child in her bedroom: unconfined, pure, idealistic, full of potential.

To finish the exercise, bring your hands to the lower belly and rest.

Further exercises for the kidneys

REFRESHING THE KIDNEYS

We start this exercise supine, lying on the back with the legs bent and feet on the ground. Maintain space under the knees – do not bring the heels too close to the buttocks. In this exercise, you will roll the pelvis forwards and backwards with each inhale and exhale.

As you inhale deeply into the belly, tip the pelvis forwards towards the coccyx. The lumbar naturally arches, lifting the kidneys. As you exhale, tip back: the pubic symphysis rolls in and down towards the bladder, the coccyx points up, the kidneys descend. Let the belly inflate and deflate naturally as you rock with each breath. The sacrum stays on the ground throughout the exercise.

Now, bring your heels closer to your buttocks, aligning them more or less under your knees. Lift your arms to the sky. On exhale, press down evenly through both feet so as to lift your hips. Allow your lower belly to hug in naturally. On inhale, roll back down to the ground. Experienced practitioners may want to engage *Moola Bandha*, the Root Lock, on the way up.

This exercise can be performed with breath retention. It is best to do this while your hips are lifted. Hold your breath at the end of your exhale for three or four seconds before rolling down with your inhale. While performing breath retention exercises, it is important not to force yourself.

Release the hold before you feel the need to. Your capacity to retain the breath will improve with regular practice, not by pushing yourself to the limits of what feels comfortable or possible.

To generate even more warmth for the kidneys, you can add a further variation. The next time you bring your hips to the ground, raise both legs, keeping the knees bent. Reach your arms forwards between your legs. Lift your head and shoulders if possible. Pull your knees back towards your ears. As you exhale, release your feet to the ground and raise your hips to continue the cycle.

SPHINX POSE VARIATION

As the Kidney meridian rises up the legs, the energy runs deep along the inner seams of the thighs, before moving into the groin and up into the torso. The meridian branches forward to meet the Conception Vessel below the navel. Another spur extends back towards the lumbar spine to meet the Governor Vessel between the second and third lumbar vertebrae. Sphinx Pose is often practised in Yin Yoga to stimulate kidney qi. Here is a variation of this practice in which we move the torso with breath.

Lie prone, on the belly, with the legs relaxed and long behind you. Release your throat, your buttocks and your ankles. Prop yourself up on your forearms, keeping the pubic symphysis on the ground. Let your belly be soft. Ideally, place the elbows under the armpits, but adjust the arms until you find a sustainable position where your ribcage feels lifted and where you can breathe comfortably. Here is the movement: turn the chest to one side, using your forearms to help you turn. Press down through your forearms, and turn to look to the side. Sometimes one shoulder will dip down. You will feel a deep stretch along the inside of the thigh, through the groin, into the inguinal area and up into the space under the ribs. As best as you can, maintain the full wingspan of your collarbones. Try not to sink down into them. If the sensation is too intense, move your elbows further apart to reduce the extension of the spine. Stay for a few breaths on each side, resting in between if needed. Repeat this exercise several times on each side for short stretches of time.

Experienced practitioners may want to build up to staying on each side for three to four minutes. If your spine extends freely, explore propping your forearms up on foam blocks or a bolster. This will deepen the sensation in your lower back and within the body. Be careful not to overstretch.

CAMEL POSE VARIATION

The Kidney meridian's journey upwards continues along the front of the chest up into the collarbones. To stimulate this section of the meridian, practise postures like Camel Pose and Crescent Pose, if they can be sustained safely. Here are two variations of upper chest postures that stimulate qi flow in the Kidney meridian along this final section on the chest.

Stand or kneel facing a wall. If you are standing, stand as close to the wall as you can, and place the pubic symphysis against the wall. If you are kneeling, bring the knees and thighs as close to the wall as you comfortably can. Place your hands against the wall, with the arms stretched upwards in a 'V'. Maintain contact between the pubic bone and the wall as you pull your heart up. Use the traction of your palms against the wall to do this. You will naturally find yourself leaning back a little. Imagine a gentle, soothing waterfall showering down on you. Avoid crunching into the back of your neck. There is no need to push the chin up or lift your gaze unless it is comfortable for your neck to do so. If your shoulders feel restricted, bend your arms a little. This exercise is a useful alternative for students who find Sphinx Pose and its variations uncomfortable. It is also useful as a transition pose into standing balances or inversions practised at a wall.

WATERFALL – RESTORATIVE POSTURE

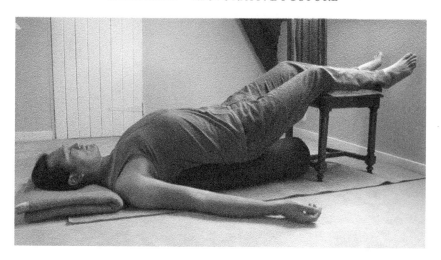

This is a supine restorative posture that will require a bolster or two thick blankets or towels. In this posture, the spine is elevated from the coccyx to the mid-thoracic. If a bolster is too high or too firm, use blankets or towels to create a level, comfortable and supportive prop to elevate this section of your spine. Your shoulders and head are resting on the ground. Your arms can be on your belly or stretched out alongside your body. You can place your legs on a chair or keep the feet on the floor. Experienced practitioners can try extending their legs on the ground. If the legs roll out too much and pinch the back, use a strap to hold the legs parallel and avoid external rotation in the hips.

Once in this posture, allow each breath to bring a wave of release to any part of the body that feels tight. You may feel energy flowing towards the head and upper chest in the first few moments in this posture. Stay present to the sensation of energy flowing from the lower belly up along the chest to the collarbones. This sensation may feel quite intense in the first few moments that you come into the posture, but it should even out after a few long breaths. If pressure continues to build to an uncomfortable level, come out of the posture, remove the props and lie flat on the floor, using a chair or the edge of a sofa to elevate your legs.

KIDNEY RECHARGE – RESTORATIVE POSTURE

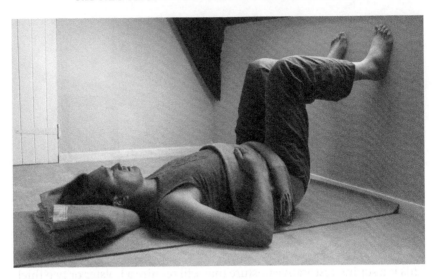

This is a deeply delicious, restorative supine posture, especially during the cooler months of the year. For this posture, you will ideally have three blankets or large towels. Fold one blanket into a rectangle. This will be used as a support for the head. Fold the second blanket lengthways to create a long, thick scarf about a foot wide. Wrap this scarf around the kidneys firmly but not too tightly. Lie on your back near a wall. Position yourself so that your feet rest comfortably on the wall with your knees bent at a 90° angle. Slide the first blanket under your head. We want to use it to create a cradle for your skull. Starting at the corners by your ears, tuck these corners under, a little at a time, until you have created a support of the correct thickness for your neck and head. Your hands can rest on your belly, with your elbows on the ground beside you. If you still feel cold, cover yourself with the third blanket.

Visualise the space of your kidneys. Imagine them as a pair of glowing, deep-blue sapphires. As you lie here breathing, imagine these sapphires becoming richer, brighter and more powerful.

Pericardium meridian

*The function of the Pericardium is to protect
the heart and regulate sexual propriety.*

Frontier Gates

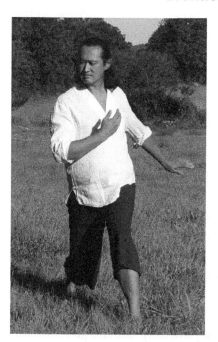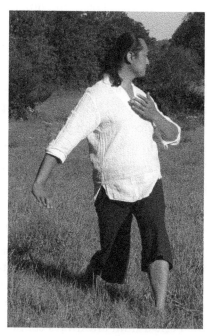

Stand comfortably and evenly. Align your palms at your heart-centre,
with the left hand over the right, aware of the *Lao Gong* point on each
hand. On exhale, press your right hand down and out to the side. As you
extend your right arm to press down and out, rotate it inwards so that the
fingers are pointing in towards the body. Keep the left hand in front of the
heart-centre. Keep your fingers close together without tensing them to
excess. Extend your right wrist, folding your hand back as much as you
can. Extending the wrist in this way stimulates the Pericardium meridian.
You may feel a light tingling sensation run down the centre of your arm
into the middle finger.

On inhale, bring the right arm back in, aligning the palms without
touching. The right hand is now on the outside, in front of the left. On
exhale, press your left palm down and out. On inhale, bring it back to

the heart-centre, aligning the palms. The left hand is now on the outside. Repeat until this movement becomes comfortable and effortless, or until the sensations running down your arms become less intense.

When you have become familiar with this movement, you can introduce the following variation: as you press one hand down, turn your head and chest in the opposite direction. One hand stays in front of the chest, soft and relaxed, the other arm is extended. Stay present to the relationship between the hands as you move. As you change arms, turn your head and chest the other way. Remember to stay aware of the hand in front of the chest.

The position of the legs can be modified for this exercise to create a more dynamic, heat-generating practice. To do this, start in a Deep Horse Stance and then progress to a lunge, making sure that you repeat the arm movements for an equal duration on each leg. For Deep Horse Stance, stand with your legs wider than your hips, but not so far that you are unable to bend your knees. Align your knees above your ankles. Your feet can turn out to a comfortable degree. From here, you can pivot on the feet to either side to perform this exercise in a lunge.

The Pericardium is the gatekeeper of the Heart. Although often likened to the bouncer at a club, the relationship is actually much subtler and more intimate. Perhaps a better analogy would be to view the Pericardium as the personal bodyguard to the Emperor. The Heart and the Pericardium are always connected physically and energetically. The Heart can be free and relaxed when the Pericardium is functioning well. Although it performs a gatekeeper role, if the Pericardium is too tightly closed off, the Heart becomes lonely, sad and deprived of joy, love and stimulation. If the Pericardium is too lax in controlling access to the Heart, the Heart can become overwhelmed and find herself unable to cope. The communication and connection between them need to be open and well lubricated in order for both to thrive.

Another way to look at this relationship is to view the Pericardium as our 'public face' and the Heart as our 'private face'. We all have both aspects, yet we remain the same person. We discern instinctively what can appropriately be made public and what is best kept private. This is the discourse between the Heart and the Pericardium. As you move deeper into the Frontier Gates exercise, stay present to the relationship between the two hands: one covering the heart space; the other opening to the world. Be aware of the different sensations as the hands move apart and then the sensations of the hands coming back towards each other. This practice can also be tuned to match your intention for the day; for example, to clear or cut off old and lingering heart connections or to welcome and nurture new relationships.

Triple Heater meridian

The function of the Triple Heater is to
regulate the three burning spaces.

Crane Arms

Stand evenly. Bring the backs of your hands to look at each other in front of the lower belly. On inhale, sweep the arms forward and out like a crane spreading its wings. Let your chest and heart expand. Roll your arms and palms to face outwards. On exhale, bring the arms back in and repeat the exercise. Observe the gentle pumping action of the chest forward and back as you sweep your arms out and in. Stay aware of the trajectory of the Triple Heater meridian running up the outside of the arms to the side of the neck. This can also be performed in Deep Horse Stance or as a variation in Tree Pose.

Wrist Rolls

Simply and slowly roll your hands, flexing and extending the wrists in a circular motion. Roll your fingers in towards you. This means your right hand will be rolling anticlockwise, and your left hand will be rolling clockwise. Start with your arms softly bent and the hands in front of the solar plexus. As you roll your hands, observe the rhythm of your breath. Stay present to any sensations moving through your fingers, your hands and your arms.

As you continue rolling your wrists, lengthen your arms down alongside your body. Remember to move and breathe slowly. If possible, after a few minutes, try pulling the fingertips into a beak as the fingers roll in.

Turn the beak inwards and downwards as the arms lengthen. As your fingers roll forward again, release the beak and soften your fingers.

A variation of this exercise is to practise these wrist rolls with the arms outstretched to the sides and moving more freely. Keep your heart-centre soft and the space on your back open. Keep your hands slightly forward of the chest and your shoulders and elbows soft and easy. Keep your feet parallel, your knees buoyant, your buttocks unclenched and your belly soft. As you start to roll your wrists, gently rock back towards your heels. As you roll your hands down, lengthen your arms back behind you. Gently rock forward so more weight is in the front of your feet. As your hands move forward, rock back into your heels.

Repeat this slowly, inhaling as you roll your hands forward and exhaling as you lengthen your arms down and back. Find a rhythm to match your breathing. Don't rock forwards or backwards so much that your body tenses. The limits are very evident: rock too far back and the abdomen and the back muscles start to clench. Rock too far forward and your toes will start to grip, your neck may tighten and your belly may harden. You want your feet to stay grounded as you rock back and forth, so avoid lifting your toes or heels as you move.

Notice the spiralling motion of your hands and arms. Notice the momentum and the inertia in each arm, and how they change while you perform this exercise. Allow your arms to move more freely as energy builds.

This is an excellent exercise for anyone experiencing blockages in the wrists and shoulders, who are consequently unable to practise postures such as Downward Facing Dog or Plank. These rotations will loosen and reawaken mobility in the wrists.

Opening Shoulders and Arms

Position your forearms in front of your face, with your fingers pointing up and your palms facing you. If possible, bring the forearms to touch. On inhale, let your arms and heart rise. If your forearms are together, keep them together as you move. On exhale, lower your arms and separate your elbows. Bring the hands behind you, rolling both arms inwards. Try to bring the backs of the hands to touch each other. Lengthen the arms back and down as much as possible. Keep the crown of your head lifted, spine tall, feet stable and knees unlocked. If the hands don't touch, don't worry. Keeping the arms rolled inward, lengthen them down behind you as far as they will go. Avoid rounding your back or sinking your head as you do this.

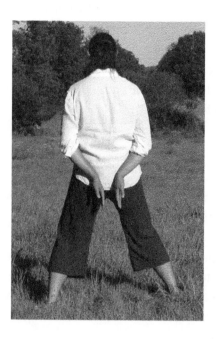

On the next inhale, raise both arms forward, bringing your forearms together as before and allowing the elbows and heart to rise. Repeat – to establish a steady rhythm for your breath and your arm movements in this exercise. When you have found a comfortable pace, introduce the following movement in the neck.

On exhale, as you move your arms down and behind you, turn your head to one side. On inhale, as your arms come forward, turn to look forward again. On the next exhale, as you lower your arms, turn your head the other way. Repeat evenly on both sides.

The direction of energy flow on this meridian is from the hands to the head. Observe any sensations rising up the side of your neck as you perform this exercise. The energy along this stretch of the Triple Heater meridian is associated with our ability to rise above life's challenges when they weigh us down. The names of energy points along this part of the body convey this beautifully: *Tian Liao* (Heavenly Bone) and *Tian You* (Heavenly Window). *Tian* means heaven. The character is derived from the image of a person reaching up to the sky. The character for *liao* (meaning bone) contains a component meaning the fluttering wings of birds. This conveys the light, active, upward movement. The character for *you* is drawn with the characters for a half of a tree and a window with light underneath. These components indicate the wisdom, teachings and discoveries that are revealed as we rise out of earthly concerns.

This exercise can be incorporated into Pyramid Pose to introduce more movement along the spine and shoulders while moving in and out of a deep forward fold.

Pumping the Triple Heater

Stand with your hands on your lower belly. On inhale, turn your palms to face upward and then bring both hands up from the lower belly to the level of your collarbones, with the palms still facing upwards. On exhale, flip your palms over and press your hands down, moving from your collarbones to the lower belly. Repeat this to establish a rhythm. As they move, keep your hands a few inches forward of your body. Your fingers point towards each other. Your shoulders and elbows stay soft and relaxed throughout.

Stay present to any sensations in your hands as you move them past your lower belly, the middle of your torso and your chest. These are the three centres of heat in the body that give the Triple Heater its name. Notice if the texture changes as you move your hands upwards and downwards. Sometimes it may feel as though your hands are moving through light mist; sometimes it may feel like your hands are moving through something denser and heavier. Repeat this movement until it feels effortless.

The next time you press your palms down, raise your heels at the same time. This is done on an exhalation. As you inhale your hands up in front of the chest, bring your heels back down to the ground. Keep the top of your head lifted and light. Your neck stays free and your throat stays spacious. Gaze into the distance. Keep your shoulders soft as you move. In addition to stimulating the Triple Heater, this movement naturally stimulates the *yin* meridians that rise along the inner legs – the Kidney meridian, the Liver meridian and Spleen meridian – all of which feed and support the Triple Heater's function and whose physical organs lie within the space governed by the Triple Heater.

Liver and Gallbladder meridians

The function of the Liver is to be in charge of planning. The function of the Gallbladder is to be responsible for judgement and decision-making.

Pivot, Twist, Push

Start in Horse Stance, with the hands at the level of your liver and arms softly bent. On exhale, pivot to the right, bending your right leg and lifting the heel of your left foot. Pull your right elbow back, keeping the arm close beside you. Make a soft fist with your right hand. Firmly, but not aggressively, press your left palm forward.

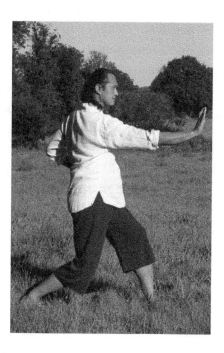

On your inhale, bring your entire body back to centre, facing forward.

On the next exhalation, pivot on your feet to turn left and repeat the movement. Explore different speeds as you pivot from side to side. Use your gaze to keep you steady. Setting your gaze on a point on the horizon will help you to maintain your balance. Stay aware of your contact with the ground through the movement of your feet, but also be aware of the distance and space ahead of you.

This exercise taps into the qualities of perspective, change, momentum and assertion, all of which relate to the Liver and Gallbladder. To make the most of this exercise, remember to keep the movement of the arms at the level of your liver and gallbladder.

Chair Pose and variations

Chair Pose and its various adaptations are strong postures for activating the Liver and Gallbladder meridians. In its simplest form, you sit back onto an invisible chair behind you. When you do this, do not push your knees forward. Keep them aligned above your ankles as much as you can. You can choose to stay higher up and keep your hands on your hips. If your legs are together, hug them into the centre line of the body as you sit back. Imagine deepening into the groin. If you are choosing to keep your legs apart, keep your feet parallel, spread your toes and press evenly down both sides of each foot. Keep the space from the crown of your head to your tailbone long and open. Do not push your chin forward or shorten the back of your neck. Do not tense your shoulders. Keep your tongue and throat relaxed, and let your gaze rest softly on the ground ahead of you.

Now, try to take a twist while in this pose. Gently turn your chest while maintaining this sitting position. Keep your spine long. If you are staying higher up, hold your elbows in front of your chest. Advanced students can sit deeper and hook the elbow outside the opposite knee.

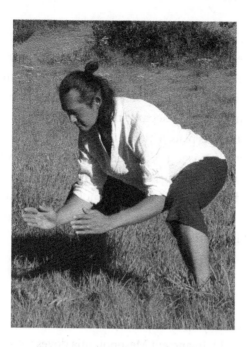

Another variation is to place the elbows against the inside of both knees, sitting deep in the pose. This is almost a squat, so take your time to build up to this.

This position applies pressure to a point on the Liver meridian, above the crease of the knee. The point is called *Qu Quan* (Crooked Spring) and is a nourishing point for the Liver meridian. The refreshment present at this point is akin to stopping for a drink at a natural spring, midway through a long hike up a mountain.

Lung meridian

*The function of the Lung is to receive the
purest qi from the heavens.*

Opening to Heaven

Start in Horse Stance, with your arms loosely hanging down beside you. On inhale, scoop your hands up in front you, crossing your forearms. Raise your arms overhead. On exhale, turn both palms out to the sides and slowly circle your arms back down. Repeat this movement slowly. Let your breath lead you through this movement. At the summit of the inhale your arms are overhead, and at the end of your exhale your arms are back down beside you. Move as slowly as you can without labouring the breath. Keep the pace of your breathing steady and slow but comfortable. This movement is similar to the Separating Clouds exercise. In Opening to Heaven, our attention is placed higher than the clouds, up in the imagined heights of heaven. This is important because the qi received by the lungs is the purest energy. Our lungs will not thrive on anything less.

I often include this exercise for longer holds in Warrior 2. The rotation in the shoulders can help to free any unconscious tension for transitions from Warrior 2 into Side Angle Pose and Triangle Pose.

Dove Spreads Wings

The dove is used to symbolise peace, love and divinity in all the major religions of the world. In ancient Mesopotamia doves were symbols for the goddess of love, sexuality and war. In this exercise, imagine your arms are the wings of a dove. Move with the intention of cultivating peace within yourself and for all life on earth.

Step your right foot forward. Open your arms wide and shift your body forward as though moving to hug someone. Keep both feet steady and both heels on the ground. Now, sweep your arms in, bringing your hands towards your chest. The palms are turned in, a palm facing each lung. As you do this, shift your body weight into the back (left) leg. Then circle your arms out to repeat the movement, shifting your weight forward again into your front (right) leg.

In this exercise, the distance between the feet can be modified depending on what feels possible for each individual. Start with a small step forward, not a deep lunge. What matters is the stability through the legs, so we can comfortably shift the body weight forwards and backwards, from one leg into the other. We want to keep both heels on the ground.

As your arms open, spread your wings wide. Spread your embrace as far as you can. As you bring your hands in, imagine yourself welcoming the dearest beings in your life into your heart. Keep your arms at the level of your shoulders: this will stimulate the Lung meridian. Repeat the exercise equally on both sides, with the left foot and right foot forward.

For advanced practitioners, this exercise can be performed in a crescent lunge or as a variation for Warrior 1.

The Liver-Lung connection

The next four exercises are designed specifically to stimulate the area connecting the Liver meridian to the Lung meridian. At the base of the ribcage, the Liver meridian goes deep into the body, weaving through the liver and both lungs. This is where it meets the deep section of the Lung meridian. The Lung meridian surfaces under the collarbone before travelling down the arm.

LIVER-LUNG EXERCISE 1

Stand in Horse Stance. Place your hands on your hips. Slowly sink into your right leg. Over the course of three or four breaths, shift more of your body weight onto your right leg. Keep the crown of your head lifted and your spine long. When you have shifted fully onto your right leg, stay for a few breaths and observe the weight and work in the right leg. On your next exhale, press down through the right foot to bring yourself back to centre. Observe the rising motion of the body initiated in the foot. When you are ready, shift your weight over onto the left leg. Move slowly. Give your left leg some time to receive the weight of your body and to stabilise. As you did before, stay for a few breaths on this leg, and when you are ready, on an exhale, press down through the left foot to bring yourself back to centre. As you repeat, notice the speed you're moving at. Notice your heartbeat. Notice the pace of your breath. Notice the muscles working in your legs. Notice also the rotation in the hips and the torso as you shift from side to side.

Now, imagine your hands are the claws of a tiger. Sense how this very suggestion may have changed the sensations in your fingertips. You may want to curl the fingertips a little to make the shape of a claw. Do not tense the hands too much, as this will restrict the flow of energy. Lengthen your arms down towards the ground, turning your palms down towards the earth as you continue to shift from one leg to the other. Your hands are like the claws of a tiger. Observe the sensations rising up your legs and down your arms.

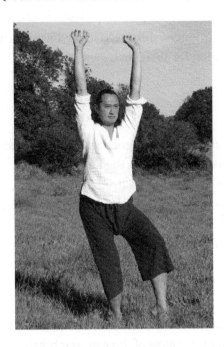

For a more challenging version of this exercise, reach your claws to the sky as you move from one leg to the other. Stay aware of the trajectory of your extremities as you move: your feet pressing into the ground; your fingers reaching to the sky. Explore how this may influence any transitions into standing balances like Warrior 3 or Eagle Pose.

LIVER-LUNG EXERCISE 2

Start in Horse Stance. In this exercise, we circle the arms at the level of the liver. To start, position your arms as you would if you were to present a tray of jewels to a queen, or if you were to present a sword to a warrior, your forearms parallel. Your elbows are softly bent, close to your ribs. On an inhale, slowly reach both arms further forward. As you exhale, circle both arms out and round behind you. Bring your hands forward again just below the ribcage, palms upward, at the level of your liver.

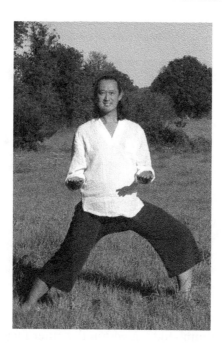

Once this movement feels comfortable, you can introduce the following movement in the legs. Rotate your legs and feet to the right as you would for Triangle Pose. On inhale, as your hands move forward from beside the ribs, bend the right knee. On exhale, as you sweep your arms out and back, press down through the right foot and lengthen the leg. Rise through the spine. Repeat evenly on both sides. Explore transitioning from here into Side Angle Pose, Triangle Pose or Half Moon Pose.

LIVER-LUNG EXERCISE 3

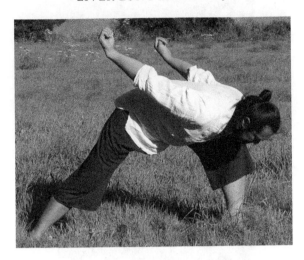

This exercise continues on from Liver-Lung Exercise 2. Start by making soft fists, with the thumb hidden within the other fingers. This is called *Zhang Wo*, a soft fist that symbolises containment, strength and potential, without force or violence. Reach your arms down beside you and slightly back. Position your legs for Warrior 2. On exhale, fold forward from the hips towards the inside of the bent leg. Keep your arms strongly raised behind you. On inhale, rise back up. As you bring yourself back up, trace the lines of energy running up the inside of the legs into the groin area, and along the inside of your arms from the soft fists to the collarbones. Stay anchored through the balls of your feet. Keep your toes relaxed. Repeat evenly on both sides. Experienced practitioners may want to try this in a Deep Horse Stance. Observe the quality of your breathing as you perform this exercise. Work to a degree where you may feel that you are generating heat, but don't push so far that you find yourself gasping for an inhale.

For advanced practitioners, this exercise could lead to Standing Wide-Legged Forward Fold, Headstand or Handstand.

LIVER-LUNG EXERCISE 4

Start in Deep Horse Stance. Raise your right arm and press your palm to the sky, with the wrist facing outwards. At the same time, press the palm of your left hand downwards. Align both hands vertically along the centre line of your body. This that means your right hand is over your head and your left hand is in front of your lower belly.

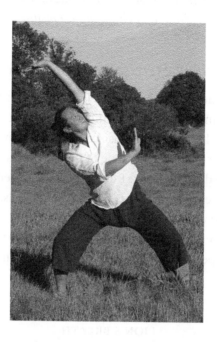

Keeping your legs steady, lean to the left, bringing your right arm with you. Like in Sparrowhawk Takes Flight, extend the left arm across your chest, under your right armpit. Press the palm of the left hand past your right armpit. Turn your head to the right, looking up to the sky. Stay for a few breaths in this position. On an inhale, bring yourself back to centre. Turn both palms to face each other and then bring them to your heart-centre. Let the left arm continue up towards the sky, and press the palm of your right hand down. Lean to the right to repeat the exercise.

As you perform this exercise, stay aware of the relationship and tension between your two hands as they press away from each other. Trace the energy rising through your legs up into your chest and your raised arm.

Sequence this exercise into poses such as Prayer Twist, Easy Twist, Revolving Triangle, Twisting Half Moon, Kneeling Warrior and Twisted Reverse Warrior.

Large Intestine meridian

*The function of the Large Intestine is to
drain and eliminate rubbish.*

Breathing exercises focusing on exhale

When the Large Intestine functions well, the dregs and waste produced
in daily life are eliminated without difficulty. Beyond the evacuation of
physical waste, the Large Intestine also controls the clearing of our mental,
emotional and spiritual rubbish. One of the best ways to encourage this
is through focused exhalations. Remember, the superficial channel of
the Large Intestine meridian ends beside the nostrils. From there, the
meridian goes down, at a deeper level in the body, into the physical organ
in the lower abdomen. As you perform the following breathing exercises,
visualise this deeper section of the meridian travelling down from the
nose to the anus.

LION'S BREATH

This exercise is performed with a long, forceful exhale. Stick your tongue
out as you exhale. If possible, turn your eyes to look up towards the centre
of your forehead. When you breathe in, relax your tongue and your eyes. If
you prefer, you can close your eyes when you inhale. Breathe in naturally.
Take a few normal, easy breaths if your breathing starts to feel strained.
Stop immediately if you feel light-headed. This is an invigorating breath
and can be woven into energetic sequences. When performed at the peak
of a class, this breath can have a very cleansing effect.

When sticking your tongue out, do not push your head, neck and
jaw forward. To open the mouth comfortably, let the jaw drop and let the
tongue extend naturally. If you feel tension at the base of the skull, you're
pushing too hard. Ease the tongue back in slightly.

HORSE BREATH

Seal your lips, softly but completely. Push the breath out through your
sealed lips making them flutter, like a horse snorting. Breathe in normally.

In a group setting, this exercise rarely fails to initiate a shared moment of laughter. Try it, enjoy it. It is an excellent way to release tension in the face. When performed in Downward Facing Dog, this exercise is an effective way to encourage the diaphragm to lift.

GRITTED TEETH

Breathe out through your teeth with the jaw closed. Keep exhaling until your breath is completely out. This will encourage the diaphragm to fully lift. Close the lips to allow the inhale to enter through the nose.

This exercise can quickly cool the body. Good times to introduce this exercise may be at the end of the class before relaxation or to start a class on a sweltering summer afternoon.

THREE-PART EXHALE

Take a long breath in without overfilling. Divide the exhalation into three parts, with a short pause between each third. It may be useful to visualise the space from the tailbone to the top of your head being full of breath. Empty the first third from the head to your heart. Pause for a second and then release the second third from your heart to your belly button. Take another short pause and then empty the rest all the way down to the base of your spine. This exercise can quickly calm the heart. It can be performed seated, supine or in a backbend (for example, Wheel Pose or the restorative posture for the kidneys, Waterfall).

Movements to stimulate the Large Intestine meridian

RESTORATIVE WRIST STRETCH

Lie on your back with your knees bent and the soles of your feet comfortably on the ground. Separate your feet, and let your thighs and knees rest against each other. Place a blanket or pillow under your head if you need one, but don't lift your head so high that your throat closes.

Lift your arms to the ceiling. Cross the right arm over the left (the right arm is now nearer your face) and then roll your thumbs out and forwards until your palms face each other. Now interlace your fingers. Keep your arms lifted toward the ceiling. Using your right hand, pull your left hand to flex your left wrist. Trace the stretch along the radial ridge from your forearm all the way to the neck. If possible, turn your head to the right as you do this. Trace the line of the meridian as it continues up your neck towards the side of your nose, paying particular attention to the space around your nostrils. After a minute or two, bring your hands and head back to centre and repeat the movement to the other side.

I like to teach this pose as a precursor to relaxation at the end of a class because it aligns with the intention to release the mind and body into rest. However, this exercise can be used at the start of a class to open the meridian and stretch the arms, shoulders and neck while seated or standing. It can also be used as a precursor to poses such as Eagle Pose and Temple Pose.

GREAT EAGLE SPREADS HIS WINGS

In this exercise, the exhalation used is Lion's Breath. If you prefer not to practise Lion's breath, you can still perform the exercise with a normal, full exhale.

Stand evenly. On inhale, raise both arms forward and then out to the sides, making a T-shape. Turn your palms to the sky. Hold the thumb and fingers of each hand close together, with the thumbs touching the index fingers. Reach your arms long. Visualise the wings of a great eagle.

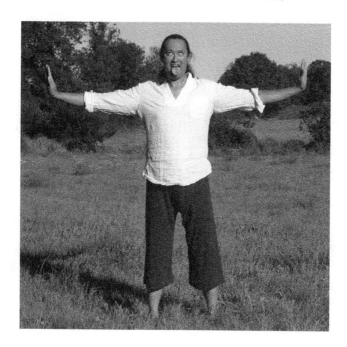

On exhale, turn your palms to press them out to the sides, pointing the fingers to the sky. On this exhale, stick your tongue out for Lion's Breath. Trace the line of the meridian from the index finger up the side of the neck to the nose. On inhale, turn the palms to the sky again. You can pause here for a breath before repeating the movement.

OLD MONK CHOPS WOOD

This is an exercise from the *Luohan Qigong* tradition.

Stand with your feet comfortably apart. Pivot both feet to the right and shift your weight into the back (left) leg. Raise your right arm and right knee. Bending your left elbow, raise your left hand to the level of your right elbow. Bring both hands down in a chopping motion. At the same time, firmly, not aggressively, stomp the right foot to the ground. When you bring the foot down, bring it down further out so that the legs are wider apart, as in Warrior 2.

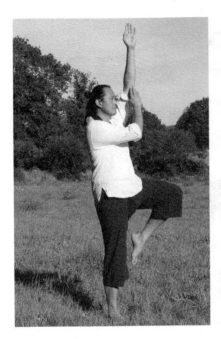 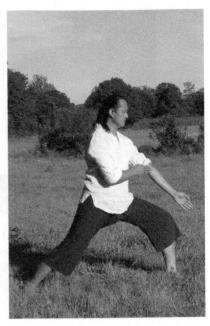

Now pivot to the left, sinking the body weight into the right leg. Pull your left leg back in to bring it up. Lift your arms, leading with the left. Bring the arms down in a chopping motion, lightly stomping the left foot to the ground. Repeat evenly on both sides.

The sharp, clear movement of the arms and the foot coming down are qualities that correspond to the finality and decisive nature of elimination.

Stomach and Spleen meridians

The function of the Stomach is to rot and ripen food. The function of the Spleen is to transform and transport nutrients throughout the body.

Exercises for the Stomach and Spleen meridians

ROLLING THE QI BALL

Unlike the Rolling Ball exercise to bring qi to the hands (see Chapter 5), this exercise is focused at the level of the stomach. The stomach churns and digests everything we take in so that it can be converted into energy.

Healthy stomach energy will provide suitable lubrication so that this process can happen smoothly. An important energy point is situated on the Stomach meridian just above the level of the navel, called *Hua Rou Men* (Gateway of Food Lubrication). *Hua* means slippery, smooth, polished. The character contains the radical for water, which indicates the importance of fluidity and hydration in this process of digestion. *Rou* is the word for meat but in this case means food. This point along the Stomach meridian, where the stomach connects to the intestines, is a critical gateway (*men*) in the digestion process. Healthy qi will enable the smooth processing and passing through of all nutrition. Hold this image in your mind as you perform this exercise.

If your hands are cold, rub them together to generate some heat before you start this exercise. Position your hands at the level of your stomach, cupping them softly as if cradling a small ball of dough. Gently knead this ball of dough, rolling and stretching rhythmically, being sensitive to sensations in your hands. It may take some time for this feeling to arrive in your hands. You will want to use a combination of rolling and stretching actions to stimulate this ball of energy in your hands. You may feel the sensation between your hands expand as you continue to massage it. Visualise the smoothness of this ball of energy between your hands. When the small ball of dough has expanded into a larger ball of energy between your hands, bring your hands to the level of your stomach, placing the energy you've generated in your hands back into your body.

Here is a variation of this exercise from the Wild Goose tradition. Bend your arms and position your hands at the level of your stomach. Your forearms form a horizontal axis from left to right. Keep your upper arms and elbows steady. Spin or twirl your hands around each other, like two paddles turning around each other along this horizontal axis. Some students find it much more natural to twirl the hands 'up and over', while some find it more natural to go 'down and under'. Either orientation is fine, but try both and observe the differences.

Notice the weight or texture as you move your hands. Find a rhythm that feels effortless and frictionless. Continue this twirling motion as you turn your torso from side to side, going as far as is comfortable to the left and then rotating slowly as far as you can to the right. Invite a sense of lightness, ease and flow to your hands and arms as you perform this exercise. To end the exercise, return to centre and place your hands on your belly, anchoring the energy back within the body.

This exercise can be used at the start of a class that focuses on core work to bring attention to the abdominal area and the deeper muscles such as the spinal erectors.

BRINGING QI TO THE CENTRE

This is one of the closing movements from the *Shibashi* second series.

Standing comfortably, bring your hands to the level of your navel. Turn your palms to face down to the ground. Circle both hands anti-clockwise three times and then clockwise three times, making the circles parallel to the ground. Move slowly and smoothly. After circling three times each way, reach both arms out to the sides and up, and then slowly press your palms down in front of the centre of your chest, returning the hands to the lower belly.

This exercise is a useful transition between standing poses such as lunges and standing twists, as it reminds the student to stay aware of and return to the centre.

OPENING TO EARTH

Stand with your feet wide apart. On inhale, sweep your arms out and up overhead. On exhale, bring the arms down in front of the body, crossing the forearms. Continue to sweep out and up again as you inhale and repeat the cycle. Keep your breath steady and slow, without labouring.

The next time you bring the arms down, bend your legs to lower yourself into Deep Horse Stance. As you sweep your arms up again, bring yourself back up. Repeat this cycle slowly and steadily. Mentally trace these lines of the Stomach and Spleen meridians as you move in the exercise: the Stomach meridian travels down the front of the body along the nipple line, and the Spleen meridian rises up the inner seam of the legs from the big toe to the armpits. Notice the spaciousness that evolves beneath your feet as you perform this exercise.

This exercise can lead to deeper hip and hamstring openers like

Garland Pose, Head to Knee Pose, Pigeon Pose, Double Pigeon Pose, Cow Facing Pose, Cobbler's Pose and Wide-Legged Seated Forward Fold.

EMPTY STANCE

The energy point on the centre of each nipple is called *Ru Zhong* (Centre of the Breast). *Ru* means to suckle. *Zhong* means the central point or hub. The character for *ru* is drawn to convey the image of birds nesting their young – a warm, safe hub where new life receives nourishment. As you perform this exercise, hold this image of being nurtured or nurturing, and of rich nourishment like that which can only be provided by a mother.

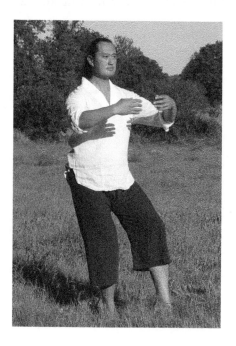

Stand evenly. Bring your hands to the level of your chest, aligning *Lao Gong* on each hand with *Ru Zhong*. Turn both thighs slightly inward, deepening into the space in your groin. Allow the space behind your sacrum to broaden. Let your back be wide and full. Let your chest be receptive and soft. Shift your weight into your left leg. Sink into your left leg to a degree that feels sustainable, without strain. You may want to turn your body 45° to the right.

Lightly lift the heel of your right foot. Keep the toes and the ball of the foot on the ground for stability. As much as possible, place your body weight on the left leg.

As you inhale, feel energy rise from the left foot up the back of your body to the top of your head. As you exhale, visualise the flow of energy moving down the front of your body, through the legs into the ground. Stay here for four or five long breaths and then return to standing evenly on both feet. When you feel ready, shift into the right leg for four or five long breaths. With practice, you can build up to ten breaths or more on each leg. While holding the pose, check that your shoulders are not tensed or hitched up and keep your elbows relaxed.

I often use this exercise in the lead up to standing or walking meditation.

Chapter 5

BRINGING QI TO THE ARMS AND LEGS

Part 1: Building qi in the hands and arms

Nyasam

This is a simple and profound practice to bring energy to the hands. In addition to improving blood circulation and flexibility of the hands, this exercise also focuses and grounds the mind. It was taught to me in a matter of minutes by Ganga, my teacher at the Krishnamacharya Yoga Mandiram in Chennai. I use this to warm my hands when I am cold, and in particular when I am about to make bread, as it brings such delightful sensitivity into my fingers for working the dough.

Start this exercise with one hand, sliding the tip of your thumb up the index finger from its base to its tip. Then roll the tip of the thumb over and onto the fingernail, so that the thumb tip folds over the fingernail of the index. Now, flick the index finger free of the thumb tip. Continue the exercise by placing the tip of the thumb at the base of the middle finger, slide the thumb tip up and roll it over the top of the middle finger and then flick. Do the same thing with the ring finger and little finger. Repeat the sequence from the index finger all the way to the little finger. You can do this one hand at a time until the movements start to feel effortless and then continue the exercise using both hands at once.

Exhale to Close Fists

This is an exercise from the *Xing Yi Quan* style of qigong. In this exercise, we use the exhale to send energy to the hands.

Begin with the hands relaxed but the fingers lightly curled in. As you breathe out, imagine your hands closing into a tight fist. Only imagine it: do not physically do it. (In some schools, this is taught by physically closing the hands into a tight fist. You can try both and adopt whichever works better for you.) The exhale becomes a vehicle to move energy down to the hands. Whether we simply imagine it or physically do it, the closing of the fists is the act of receiving the energy that we send down to the hands.

There are many arm positions used in this practice, but the following five positions are the ones that I have found to be most efficient, safe and sustainable for my students.

First position: With the arms down alongside the body, not so far back that your shoulders start to tense nor so far forward that your back starts to round.

Second position: Reach both arms forward, parallel to the ground and parallel to each other, with the palms looking at each other.

Third position: Arms opened out to the sides, parallel to the ground, with the palms facing forward.

Fourth position: Start from the third position and, without rolling or turning the arms, bend the elbows to bring your thumbs towards the sides of your head. The hands do not touch your head. The upper arms stay level with the ground.

Fifth position: Circle the hands down from the fourth position to hold them just in front of the belly, with the palms facing upwards. The elbows are comfortably bent, and the hands are an inch or two forward of the body and from each other.

Opening the Chest

This is the second movement from the *Shibashi* second series.

Opening the Chest is a deceptively simple movement that stimulates the lungs and energises the arms and upper chest. In this exercise, both arms extend forward up to horizontal and then out to the sides, making a

T-shape. This is done on one long inhale. On exhale, we release the arms down to the sides.

The position of the hands and, consequently, the rotation in the shoulders are important. As you raise the arms, the palms face each other. Keep a comfortable amount of space under your armpits as the arms come up. Keep the shoulders relaxed and elbows unlocked. As the arms go out to the sides, turn the palms to face upwards. Don't push your chest forward as the arms move out. Keep the heart-centre soft, and let your breath fill the back of your body. The palms turn down as you release the arms down. This can be done while standing evenly on both feet or with the legs in a lunge.

Holding Up the Sky

In this exercise, we hold our hands over our head, with the palms turned up toward the sky and fingers pointing in towards each other. Let the palms be soft and receptive, allowing both hands to receive the warmth of the sun. The elbows can be kept softly bent and the shoulders relaxed. Position your gaze softly skyward.

For a more dynamic variation, reach both arms straight up and press the palms to the sky. In both variations, turn the hands so that the fingers point in towards each other.

This exercise can raise the cardiac rhythm and warm the body relatively quickly, so beginners should take a progressive approach, starting perhaps with 30 seconds, extending to three minutes, then to five minutes with regular practice.

In some traditions, this is taught with the face turned sharply to the sky, with the front of the throat stretched long. Be sure to warm up the neck if you are attempting this variation, and be careful not to crunch the back of the neck. Try this in seated, kneeling or lunge postures.

Dragon Extends His Claws

To begin this exercise, the arms are down alongside the body and the hands in soft fists. On inhale, lift both hands to the level of the heart, with the palms down and knuckles facing forward, as you would if you were lifting a pail of water. On exhale, open your hands and press the palms forward, keeping the arms level with the ground. Imagine your hands transforming from soft fists into the claws of a dragon. Once the arms are fully extended, bring them back down beside you. Repeat.

As you bring your hands up, keep your shoulders soft and your jaw relaxed. As you press your hands forward, imagine the qualities you wish to carry in these claws of yours. You may be familiar with the way that cats extend their claws sometimes, just for a good stretch. This is the attitude we want to bring to this extension of claws: one of comfort and opening, not one of aggression. This is a powerful exercise for stimulating the Kidney meridian when practised in Deep Horse Stance.

Rolling Ball

This exercise is taught in many different styles of qigong. While each style brings with it some variation, I cannot say that one is better than another. The most commonly used instruction is to move your arms as though you are rolling a large ball in between both hands, so let us start there. Bring your attention to both your hands as they move. Roll the ball in a forward motion, with the palms facing one another. The hand moving forward will naturally be a little higher; the hand drawing back will be lower.

An image that many of my students find useful for this exercise is that of the ball-return system in a bowling alley. After a ball is rolled down the lane to (hopefully) knock down a few pins, the ball is brought back to the bowler on a conveyor-belt system under the lane. As in a bowling alley, the to and fro is constant while the game is in motion. Unlike the bowling alley machinery, we want this process to be smooth and steady, not loud and clunky.

Start with your arms bent beside you. Pull the elbows back so that the hands are beside the lower ribs. On an exhale, press one hand forward, 'pushing' the ball forward. On inhale, draw your hand back towards the side of the ribcage. The other hand now presses forward. As your hand moves back towards you, the palm faces up, staying open and soft.

As you move, keep your elbows softly bent, your palms soft and receptive and your shoulders relaxed. There is no need to fold your wrist deeply or tense the shoulders. As you move your arms and hands in this circular, forward-and-back motion, don't raise your hands too high. I often see students raising their hands to the level of their face or even above their head. There is nothing inherently wrong with that, but raising the arms can have the effect of shifting the energy up into the head, neck and shoulders rather than focusing the flow into the arms and hands.

Although this exercise may appear repetitive, take time to establish a rhythm with your breath. Explore each cycle with curiosity. As the spine will naturally and gently twist on its axis during this exercise, you may find energy and warmth spreading through the body, not just into the arms and hands.

Cloud Hands

In this exercise, imagine your hands swirling in a soft circular shape amidst light, fluffy clouds or morning mist. Start with one hand. Draw your hand up in front of the centre line of your torso, with the palm stroking upward to face the heart-centre and the elbow bending. Keep your shoulder relaxed and elbow down. Continue the arc to turn your arm out to the side, rotating it so that the palm faces forwards, and roll it out to the side and down, creating a soft circular motion. Repeat a few times to establish the movement and a soft rhythm. Now, do the same with the other hand. The hand ascends in front of the chest and then turns out to roll down. The shoulder and elbow stay easy and relaxed. Repeat until this feels comfortable and effortless in each arm.

Now start moving both hands at once to make alternating circles. Raise the first hand. As this hand reaches the apex of the circle and prepares to come back down, start to move the other hand. Don't get too hung up on precision here. What matters is to start with one hand and then bring in the other. Do it slowly so that you can pay full attention to the one hand as it comes up and then to the other hand as the cycle starts on the other side.

I see many students wanting to progress too quickly to moving both hands at once, and losing themselves in the struggle for coordination. This misses the point of the exercise, which is to allow each hand its moment of basking in your full, undivided attention. For how often do we give time to care for and cultivate energy within our hands? Simply look at each of your hands – one and then the other – with love, gratitude and a simple intention for them to remain in good health. The focusing of attention on this one hand is what channels energy to it. This is the best reason not to introduce the movement of both hands too quickly. If I see students struggling to coordinate both hands, I encourage them simply to repeat the exercise on one hand for three to five minutes and then do the same with the other hand, without feeling any pressure to move both arms at once.

Fisherman Casts His Net

The Chinese word for fish (*yu*) is a homonym of the word for abundance, pronounced *yu*. It also sounds like the word for jade (yes, you guessed it, also pronounced *yu*). It follows that fish are regarded as symbols of abundance, prosperity and wealth. In this exercise, we visualise a fisherman casting his net to catch fish, and it is useful to bear these symbols in mind because they suggest the optimism and the abundance of energy that we want to cultivate through this practice.

In this exercise, we simply sweep both arms from one side to the other, in the same way that we would cast a fishing net into the water. Going from the left to the right, your left hand is lower, approximately at the level of the hip, and the right hand is at the level of the chest. As you sweep the arms across to the right, the field of energy extends, like the net, beyond the physical limits of the arms. Visualise the trajectory of the net that you are casting into the water. If we throw it too far, we risk losing our balance and may fall in with it. If we don't throw it far enough, the net will not spread to its full extent and the potential catch is reduced. When you move from the right to the left, switch the position of the arms, meaning that the right arm is lower and the left arm is higher.

Feel the weight of the net in your hands. Feel the release of that weight as you cast the net out. Visualise the net spreading perfectly in a circle as it falls into the water. These images provide the general form of the movement, but in the exercise, we move slowly and continuously from side to side.

Stay firmly grounded through your feet and legs. If you are doing this seated, keep your sit bones in steady contact with your seat throughout the exercise but sit forward in the chair so that you are not slumped back. The movement of the arms is identical to the movement used when standing. Don't force the wrists or lock the elbows. Allow your body to follow the gentle side-to-side motion, but keep your legs supple and stable, with both feet grounded throughout the exercise. At the end of this exercise, bring your arms back down and pause to observe the inertia of the movement, paying attention to any sensations in the arms, head and face.

Hook and Lift

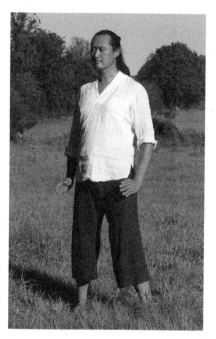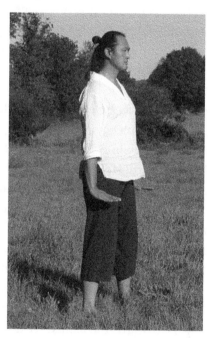

Here are two similar exercises that I have bundled together as one, because the dynamics of the movement in them are similar. In both these exercises, we extend the wrist to draw energy into the hands. In Hook, we draw the thumb side of the hand up, pulling the thumb towards the elbow, shortening the radial tendon and extending the ulnar tendon. In Lift, we turn the hand back at the wrist to press the palm to the ground, stretching the palmar tendon, shortening the extensors on the back of the hand. It is useful to know these two movements well, as they are useful exercises for students with limited wrist mobility or injury.

Let's start with Hook. I have isolated this hand movement from a movement within the *Shibashi* second series called Searching for a Needle in the Bottom of the Ocean. You can perform this exercise one arm at a time to begin with. Once you are familiar with it, perform the exercise in both arms at the same time.

Start with your arms alongside your body, with the palms turned to face the side of your legs. Stay tall through your spine, avoiding any temptation to sink or round forward as you begin to move. Bring your attention to your shoulders. Imagine a bit more space in your shoulder joints, in your elbows, wrists and in between the bones in your hands. Imagine your arms growing longer as a result of this increased spaciousness all the way through them. Imagine your fingers lengthening down towards the ground, into the earth below your feet. Now, keeping your fingers softly together, hook your hands forward. This means lifting the thumb side of the hand, shortening the radial tendon. Stay for a breath or two and then release by simply letting the hand drop, allowing your arms to completely relax or go limp. Repeat slowly. Imagine your arms reaching deep into the earth, or deep into the ocean, and then hook the hand forward. Hold here for a few breaths and then release. Stay present to the weight or buzzing in the hands after you release from the hold.

In the alternative version of this exercise, Lift, we take time to establish attention in the shoulders and arms, just as we have been doing for Hook. Let your arms hang by your sides, but this time with the backs of the hands facing forwards and the thumbs next to your thighs. Imagine the arms growing long, reaching deep into the earth or into a body of water. In this exercise, keep the fingers long and held together as you lift the fingers forward. The palms face down. Here, we want to imagine that we are lifting something on the back of the hands, like a little pebble. We do not want to push or press downwards, so, if at all possible, try lifting the fingertips. This will stretch the palmar tendon even more, so be gentle as you approach this exercise. After a few breaths here, let the hands drop, allowing the imaginary pebble on the back of your hands to plop into the water or onto soft earth. Repeat slowly. Notice the energy flowing into the hands after a few minutes of performing this exercise.

Embrace the Void

This exercise is taught in many martial arts and *Zhan Zhuang* (standing qigong) practices as one of five foundational poses.

Stand comfortably. Hold your arms out in front of you, gently rounded, with the palm of each hand aligning approximately with the upper edge of the pectoral muscle on the same side. The elbows are softly bent, and the shoulders are relaxed and not lifted. Keep your chest soft, and focus your breathing in the back of the ribcage rather than in your chest or belly. Hold for three to five minutes, or longer if it feels appropriate for your body. When you release your arms after this exercise, observe the flow of energy into the hands. Many of my students say that their hands feel larger after performing this exercise. This exercise is also a tonic for the lungs.

Expand to the Universe

In this exercise, we expand our curiosity and generosity beyond our immediate surroundings into the unknown fringes of the universe.

Stand comfortably and open your arms as though you are going to give someone a huge hug. In this exercise, though, we want to embrace more than one person. Instead, we extend our embrace to the furthest corners of the universe and include all within it.

Hold your arms slightly forward of your chest, allowing the space behind your shoulders to stay comfortably rounded and full. Keep your shoulders relaxed and easy. Do not pull your arms too wide apart and do not push your armpits forward. The arms are ideally at the level of the armpits, but if this is a struggle for the shoulders, hold the arms a little lower. What matters most is to find a sustainable position as you hold your arms out in readiness. Keep your elbows soft and your knees buoyant. Your chest stays soft and receptive.

Now, expand your sensory receptivity beyond the physical limits of your body, beyond the limits of the room you are standing in, beyond the street you are on, including everything within your radius. Expand your field of awareness slowly and gradually. If you start to feel overwhelmed or start to lose your anchor to the ground, reel it back in and work within what feels available and possible. Gradually, with time and practice, expand your sensory receptivity beyond the bounds of the planet, into space. No one knows where the limits of this universe truly lie, so let your imagination take you there.

A potent variation to this practice is to include the following breathing exercise whilst holding this posture.

Let the inhale enter through the left palm and travel through to your heart-centre, and then send the exhale through your right arm and out through your palm. Visualise this loop extending to the unknown frontiers of the universe and then return as an inhale into the palm of your left hand and out again through the right. If you are new to this, start with three to five minutes, or less if that is what feels possible. To close this practice, bring one hand to the heart and the other to the lower belly. Let your inhale fill your chest and then send the exhale into the belly. When you feel sufficiently back in your body, release your arms.

Funnel to the Earth

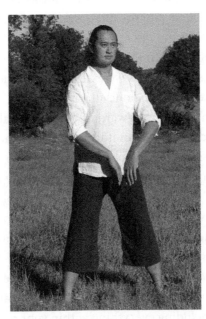

In this exercise, we hold the arms in front of the belly to make the shape of a funnel.

The forearms are directed at a diagonal down towards the pelvic region to form the funnel shape. Rotate your arms so that the backs of the hands look at each other. The shoulders and elbows are relaxed. Maintain a natural space between the hands, and between your arms and the body. Imagine water flowing down the arms and dripping off your fingertips into the earth below. Keep the crown of your head aligned to the sky, breathing freely. Observe the sensations flowing down your arms into your hands and beyond.

Part 2: Moving qi to the legs

Deep Horse Stance

This is similar to Horse Stance, but involves sitting deeper with your feet wider apart. The legs are turned out to a comfortable degree, with the feet aligned under them. Although this posture is frequently held for an extended period of time, we should not approach it with the mindset of challenging our limits of endurance. This posture stimulates warmth and raises energy up the body from the legs. It can quickly tip from being energising into being tiring. Like frying an egg, if you don't leave it on the heat long enough, it will not be cooked. If you leave it too long, the outcome is inedible and you've wasted energy along the way.

This is a useful posture to practise in movement, in conjunction with the arm and hand exercises. Building energy in the legs can be a good way to lead into standing balance postures like Tree Pose, Half Moon Pose, Warrior 3, Eagle Pose and Dancer's Pose.

Sink Back

This movement is evident in many moving martial arts. The action of sinking into the back leg frees the front leg to lift, kick or swing at an opponent. The effectiveness of the movement in the lifted leg depends, of course, on the stability of the back leg, which we will call the standing leg. The practice of sinking back into one leg is not to build balance for standing on one leg, although this could be a useful outcome. The practice allows us to build strength in one leg at a time while remaining stable and grounded.

Start evenly on both feet. Simply shift your weight onto one leg. Bend the standing knee very slightly. Align the crown of your head, your shoulders and hips over the standing foot. Your hands can be on your hips. Lightly lift the heel of the free foot, keeping the toes on the ground. Stay here and breathe slowly. Notice any tension throughout your body that could be released: your face, throat, mouth, jaw, shoulders. Do what you can to be as comfortable as possible while maintaining your focus on the standing leg and on the feeling of your body weight sinking down into it. The torso may naturally turn towards the free leg. Stay for a duration that seems appropriate for you and then return to centre to rest for a few moments before repeating the practice on the other leg. Try adding arm positions such as Holding Up the Sky, Expand to the Universe and Embrace the Void to add variety to this exercise.

Heel Drops

This quick exercise is particularly useful when there is a need to come back down to earth, to reconnect with the body and the ground beneath us. This exercise is not recommended for anyone with recent spinal injuries.

Stand comfortably, with your knees soft. On inhale, send the balls of the feet into the earth so that the whole body lifts and the heels leave the ground. On exhale, let your heels drop back down to the ground. Try not to control the descent. Let gravity do the work. Simply let the body drop back down onto the heels. Only use appropriate force when you do this, so that you do not strain your knees or jar your spine with the impact.

Heel Drops have the effect of pulling down any excessive rising qi, reinforcing our connection to the earth through our legs. As you perform this exercise, look out for any tendency to 'hold on' or for any hesitation when it comes to allowing the body to drop. If balance is a challenge, place your hands on a wall or the back of a chair whilst performing this exercise.

Mischievous Boy Kicks His Leg

This is a movement from the *Shibashi* second series.

Start with your hands on your hips. On inhale, shift onto your right leg, and bend and lift your left leg. On exhale, extend your left leg as you would to stop a ball rolling towards you. At the same time, bend your right knee. The left foot is barely off the ground. On inhale, come back up, lifting the left knee, and exhale to return to the starting position. Repeat the exercise standing on the left leg.

Pace this movement appropriately. There is no need to push yourself to move too slowly, and moving too fast in an exercise like this can often cause more tension. Maintain ease throughout the torso up to the head as you move. Try not to crouch forward or tighten your shoulders. Keep your gaze on the horizon; this will hold you steady. Perform this exercise between three and six times on each leg.

Holy Crane Worships the Moon

This is a movement from the *Shibashi* second series.

The movement in the legs here is similar to making a curtsey. You cross one leg behind the other, bend the knees and sink the body down. In this exercise, we alternate the legs: cross the right leg behind the left first and sink down. On inhale, rise up, cross the left behind the right and sink down on exhale. The gaze is softly downward in reverence.

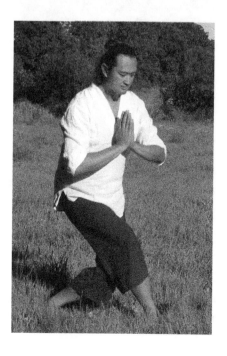

As you begin this exercise, place the palms together in front of the chest. Once you have established a rhythm and ease in the leg movements, you can introduce the arm movement. On inhale, as you rise up, circle the hands outward and upward until the palms touch overhead. On exhale, as you sink down, bring the hands back down to the chest. Repeat.

There are subtle differences if you place the weight on the back leg rather than the front leg when sinking down. Try both and explore which works better for you. I have practised and taught both versions and they are equally effective in charging and warming the legs. Some students report that rising up feels steadier when the weight is over the back leg, while others report that shifting the weight from one leg into the other makes coordination of the arms, legs and breathing during this exercise more complicated.

Pressing Air

This is from the Wild Goose series of exercises.

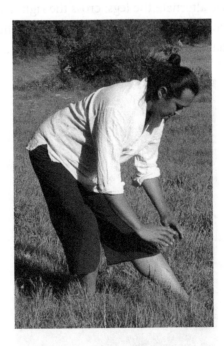

Step the left foot forward, keeping the body weight back on the right leg. Lean forward towards the left leg, lightly bending the right knee. Hover your hands on either side of the left knee, with the palms facing down-ward. Slowly press down the hands three times, moving them from the knee towards the ground. After three repetitions come back up. Change legs and repeat the exercise.

Chapter 6

INSPIRATIONS FOR SEQUENCING

For a teacher of yoga or qigong, sequencing a class can be rewarding, educational and challenging. Each sequence is an experiment and an invitation for the students to respond.

During my own early years as a teacher, I was anxious about each class sequence, wanting everything to be creative yet also exactly 'right' and 'perfectly' balanced. I have learnt that it is easy to over-engineer a sequence and so to end up disconnected from the group energy present in the room. Experience has taught me to follow my intuition and take cues from the interactions in the room as inspiration for sequencing each class.

Sequencing becomes more effortless and enjoyable with time and regular practice, but it is still important that you, as a teacher, stay refreshed and resourced. This chapter offers you some theories drawn from Chinese medicine and qigong philosophy, for you to use as material in your personal brainstorming. Experiment with them, and enjoy what you discover in the process.

Part 1: The Five Elements

In Chinese culture, there are Five Elements (*wuxing*): Metal (*jin*), Wood (*mu*), Water (*shui*), Fire (*huo*) and Earth (*tu*). They each exist in relationship to the other four and cannot be separated out of this cycle to take meaning in isolation. All the facets of human life – the physical form, the stages of life and the way a life is lived – are reflected in these Five Elements, and all five are present in nature and within us. This is how the twelve meridians relate to each of the Five Elements:

- Metal: Lung and Large Intestines

- Wood: Liver and Gallbladder

- Water: Kidneys and Bladder

- Fire: Heart, Small Intestine, Pericardium and Triple Heater

- Earth: Stomach and Spleen.

There are two kinds of relationship between these elements: the first is one of nourishment and unconditional support, the way an archetypical mother would nurture her only child. The second kind of relationship is one of respect and restraint, akin to the relationship between a stern grandmother and her precocious grandchild.

Mother and Child
Wood feeds Fire
Fire creates Earth
Earth creates Metal
Metal holds Water
Water feeds Wood

Grandmother and Grandchild
Fire melts Metal
Metal chops Wood
Wood covers Earth
Earth dams Water
Water douses Fire

While each of the Five Elements warrants a book of its own, in this chapter we will only consider how, both individually and collectively, they provide rich inspiration for sequencing yoga and qigong classes. In the Further Study section you will find some of my favourite texts on this subject. The best way to understand the Five Elements, however, is to spend time in and with nature, observing, playing and participating in its evolution and natural patterns.

Below is a concise description of how each element expresses itself when balanced and when out of balance. Use these as inspiration, as an underlying intention or as a point of departure for the tone and movement for your class.

METAL

Expressions in nature	Mountains, rocks, sand, precious stones, crystals, minerals, gases, autumn, sunset, west, rotting, decomposition, dryness, decay, the colour white
Expressions in the human body	Lungs, large intestine, skin, body hair, nose
Meridians and their functions	Lung: to receive the purest qi from the heavens Large Intestine: responsible for drainage and elimination
Emotions, behaviours and attitudes	Inspiration / Breathing / Defined Grief / Weeping / Precious Excellence / Falling / Fatherly Heaviness / Dropping / Protective Decline / Holding on / Aloof Authority / Release / Unrealistic Respect / Detoxify / Stubborn Idealism / Forgive / Transcendent Attachment / Receive / Treasured Enlightenment / Pray / Bitter Perfectionism / Honour / Unwashed Minimalist / Dream / Lacklustre Purity / Regret / Sparkling Divinity / Loss / Hollow Futility / Resignation / Clogged Emptiness / Gratitude / Ritualistic
Useful practices	Meditation and chanting Breathing exercises Decluttering Finding creative or spiritual inspiration through art, reading, music or travel

SAMPLE CLASS SEQUENCE

Exercise	Rationale
Breathing exercises, seated or standing	Establish breath as a channel for physical and spiritual inspiration
Great Eagle Spreads His Wings	Stimulate the Lung meridian
Downward Facing Dog with Horse Breath	Encourage the diaphragm to lift more fully Warm muscles in the arms, shoulders and back
Sun Salutations	Warm the body
Warrior poses	Awaken the Father archetype
Cobra/Locust Pose/Camel Pose	Stretch inhale, open ribcage
Plank and Side Plank	Activate the arms and the meridians along the inner and outer arms
Side Angle Pose	Stimulate Liver-Lung connection
Core work	Earth element strengthens Metal element
Arm balances	Require precision and a willingness to fail
Opening to Heaven, Opening to Earth	Return to the wonder of breath, and a reminder of where we stand between heaven and earth
Bridge Pose	Encourage the diaphragm to lift more fully
Knees to Chest Pose	Press the breath down and out
Supine Twists	Release the spine for seated meditation
Seated meditation with guided visualisation	Connect with inner space, transcend the mundane

WOOD

Expressions in nature	All plant life, seeds, the colour green, sunrise, east, wind, springtime
Expressions in the human body	Liver, gallbladder, tendons, ligaments, eyes, nails
Meridians and their functions	Liver: planning Gallbladder: judgement and decision-making
Emotions, behaviours and attitudes	Growth Eagerness Competitiveness Birth Assertiveness Decisiveness Rebirth Flexibility Speed Anger Upwards and Focus Change outwards New plans Action Shouting New directions Beginnings Resentment Angular Perspective Sourness Twisty Hope Thrust Curly Courage Vigour Youthful Justice Rhythm Free Benevolence Momentum Persistent Warrior-like Fertility Exuberant
Useful practices	Refreshing old routines Making a new plan and putting it into action Engaging in any physical activity that requires movement Resting your eyes

SAMPLE CLASS SEQUENCE

Exercise	Rationale
Supine Twist Happy Baby Pose Seated Twist and side stretches	Release spine, stimulate lumbar and thoracic area where Liver and Gallbladder meridians criss-cross Sequence starts on the ground and then rises progressively
Standing Forward Fold, leading to Sun Salutations	Mimic the rise of flora from the ground up to the sun
Triangle Pose, Side Angle Pose Warrior 2, into Liver-Lung Exercises 3 and 4 Crescent Lunge into Pivot, Twist, Push Chair Pose with twist and then Prayer Twist	Focus on lines of the Wood element meridians up and down the legs, and across the waist Frequent changes of direction Trajectory is upwards and outwards
Kneeling Warrior	Once warm, deeper work into the psoas muscle to stimulate the deep path of the Liver meridian from the thighs into the genitals
Standing balance postures: Tree Pose, Eagle Pose, Warrior 3, Half Moon Pose	Emphasise strength that comes through flexibility, vulnerability and perspective
Old Monk Chops Wood	In movement, it is a great transition exercise to mix with standing balance postures From an elemental perspective, some Metal to rebalance any excess Wood
Plank, Side Plank, Forearm Plank	Build core strength for inversions
Forearm Balance or Headstand	Strong inversions for advanced students A change of perspective
Shoulderstand	Counter-pose for Headstand Also a change of perspective
Seated Wide-Legged Forward Fold Pigeon Pose Supine Twist Relaxation	Deep, calm stretches to stimulate the Liver, Kidney and Bladder meridians As we slow down towards the end of class, we introduce silence and stillness (aspects of the Water element) to nourish the Wood element

WATER

Expressions in nature	Water, springs, streams, rivers, lakes, oceans, rain, mist, clouds, dew, ice, frost, the colours blue and black, winter, north, cold, salt, Antarctica
Expressions in the human body	Bladder, kidneys, bone, bone marrow, ears, head hair
Meridians and their functions	Kidney: governs reproduction and stores *jing* Bladder: controls the flow and storage of water
Emotions, behaviours and attitudes	Mystery Cooling Elusive Ancestry Sinking Deep Survival instinct Flowing Ambitious Endurance Groaning Pure Willpower Cleansing Risky Darkness Overflowing Clever Rest Deafening Lubricated Introspection Still Versatile Fear Stagnant Soft Purpose and drive Frozen Silent Death Escapist Saturated Philosopher Suspicious Fearless Wisdom Saturated Indefatigable Shapeless Unsettled
Useful practices	Hydrate appropriately Sleep, rest or spend time alone, in silence, without too much stimulation or activity Swim or be in water Study family history Practise listening without responding

SAMPLE CLASS SEQUENCE

Exercise	Rationale
Refreshing the Kidneys	Deep rest of at least 15 minutes to allow any adrenaline to dissipate
Supine Twist	Awaken the body and spine
Cobra or Locust Pose	Open the chest, focusing on the section of the Kidney meridian on the front ribs
Sphinx Pose with twist variation	Stimulate the *Ming Men* point on the lumbar spine The twist variation stimulates the Kidney meridian where it rises from the lower abdomen into the chest
Standing Forward Fold	Stimulate the Bladder meridian
Sun Salutations	Warm the body
Wild Goose sequence for kidneys	Stimulate the kidneys
Pyramid Pose	Stimulate the Bladder meridian
Twisting Triangle to Warrior 3 and then to Twisting Warrior 3 or Standing Splits	Stimulate both the Bladder and Kidney meridians Standing balances build strength in the bones Encourage students to dig deep for the drive to keep going through stronger sequences
Wide-Legged Standing Forward Fold	Cool the head and warm the heart, while stimulating the Bladder meridian Also provides a comfortable pause in the flow
Handstand	Fear is often the main barrier for this pose Practise safely
Lizard Pose and then Supported Splits	Deeper work into the hamstrings and psoas
Garland Pose and then Crow Pose Seated Twists and then Side Crow Pose	Bring the sequence closer to the ground Build stability and strength in the arm bones Again, encourage students to find the willpower to keep going, and to face fear of failing in some advanced arm balances
Bridge Pose or Wheel Pose	Stimulate Kidney meridian
Shoulderstand and Plough Pose Waterfall or Yoga Nidra	Cooling and deeply calming

FIRE

Expressions in nature	The sun, fire, the colour red, heat, south, summer, soot, ash
Expressions in the human body	Heart, small intestine, pericardium, blood vessels, tongue
Meridians and their functions	Heart: governor of the blood, home of the spirit, ruler of awareness Small Intestine: to separate the pure from the impure Pericardium: to protect the heart Triple Heater: responsible for the circulation of qi, blood, fluids and heat
Emotions, behaviours and attitudes	Spirit Heat Extrovert Desire Warmth Childlike Pleasure Expressiveness Light Vulnerability Passion Playful Laughter Silliness Fun Love Maturity Unlovable Joy Chaos Sweaty Sex Expansion Dehydrated Stimulation Addiction Enthusiastic Intensity Excess Limp Relationship Affection Radiant Communication Union Unstable Imagination Climax Kind Harmony Drama Generous Illumination Boundaries Flirtatious Understanding Magic Bubbly
Useful practices	Socialise, meet friends, make new acquaintances, be involved in a group activity Make love, flirt, tease Engage the sense of touch through manual activities like gardening, pottery, sculpting, massage, painting or drawing Find opportunities to laugh by watching or listening to comedy, reading or talking with people Allow the inner child to emerge through playfulness and silliness Make time to talk to loved ones, exchanging thoughts, ideas, feelings and secrets Be in the sun or in physical heat, for example in a sauna or steam room

SAMPLE CLASS SEQUENCE

Exercise	Rationale
Breathing exercises such as Kapalabhati and Anuloma Viloma, followed by Sun Salutations	Ignite heat in the body through *pranayama* and then warm the muscles with Sun Salutations
Crescent Lunge with Frontier Gates Golden Rooster Shakes His Wings Rolling Ball Temple Pose Small Intestine Exercises 1 and 2 Dragon Extends His Claws	A mix of movements to stimulate the Heart, Small Intestine, Pericardium and Triple Heater meridians These exercises include specific movements to bring qi to the hands and arms because all four Fire element meridians run through the hands, the arms and the shoulders
Warrior poses with lunge twists Plank, Side Plank or Forearm Plank Seated Twist and Table Pose	After a period of standing movements, reintroduce strong movement in the legs and torso to increase heat
Prone backbends: Cobra, Locust Pose, Bow Pose, Upward Facing Dog	Water + Fire = Alchemy! These backbends generate heat, and stimulate the Kidney meridian and the Fire element meridians in the arms
Preparatory poses for Handstand or Forearm Balance leading to full pose	Peak posture: a climax to the heat and energy that has been generated
Expand to the Universe	Once the heart is warm, it can be expansive, generous and magnanimous Radiate love to our wider community and all life forms
Dropbacks, Bridge Pose, Wheel Pose, Shoulderstand or some self-practice	A fire only stops once all fuel has been exhausted Offer a few choices of finishing poses for those who still have some juice to keep going Encourage creativity and playfulness
Seated in Hero's Pose for Microcosmic Orbit meditation or relaxation with heart-themed visualisation	The ambers of a fire continue to smoulder deep within Turn the attention inwards

EARTH

Expressions in nature	Planet Earth, soil, the colour yellow, humidity, central point, navel		
Expressions in the human body	Stomach, spleen, flesh, muscles, lips		
Meridians and their functions	Stomach: rots and ripens food Spleen: transforms and transports nutrients		
Emotions, behaviours and attitudes	Intention	Singing	Fragrance
	Sympathy	Nurturing	Obsession
	Support	Sharing	Manipulation
	Understanding	Grounding	Satisfaction
	Abundance	Steadying	Martyrdom
	Substance	Stabilising	Wealth
	Security	Encouraging	Sweetness
	Home	Welcoming	Ripeness
	Family	Churning	The nipple
	Material things	Pulling down	Harvest
	Transformation	Feeding	Mental agility
	The Mother	Belonging	Appetite
	Control	Gathering in	Overthinking
	Digestion	Circular	Slow
Useful practices	Self-care: get a massage; rest or pamper yourself		
	Eat healthily and appropriately		
	Practise self-acknowledgement		
	Do one thing at a time; do not take on too many tasks at once		
	Set clear intentions		
	Set clear boundaries		
	Ask for help when needed, and accept help when offered		

SAMPLE CLASS SEQUENCE

Exercise	Rationale
Empty Stance Opening to Earth Rolling the Qi Ball Pumping the Triple Heater Bringing Qi to the Centre Funnel to the Earth	Open with slow movements, like the way that Earth moves Bring attention to the immediate moment, location, breath, physical posture and thought Draw energy to the centre of the body Incorporate some Fire exercises into an Earth sequence to nourish the Earth element
Sun Salutations Boat Pose Table Pose Locust Pose	Warm the body, with awareness of where the body touches the ground Use postures that emphasise a rising from and sinking down to the ground
Seated Twists Camel Pose Gate Pose Twists on hands and knees	Practise postures that use central points such as the spine and navel as an anchor point, and track the trajectory away from the anatomical 'centre', and the return to this 'centre' as you release from the pose
Downward-facing relaxation pose on bolsters	Allow as much contact as possible between the front body and the bolsters, blankets and the ground – this will bring comfort to and tone these parts of the body Allow the body to sink down

Part 2: Seasonal transitions

As a gardener, nothing I do today is for tomorrow. Everything I do in the garden is to improve the outcome in the weeks and months ahead. The investments made now will yield rewards in future seasons, but I must wait for the change to happen. Trees and shrubs are pruned to influence spring flowering and fruiting. Some seeds are sown before the ground freezes to give them the necessary trigger to sprout when the sun warms the earth in due course. Incubating within the expression of each season are the kernels of that which is to come.

The transition from one season into the next is expressed as a Mother-Child relationship between each of the Five Elements. One gives life to the other.

Mother and Child
Wood feeds Fire
Fire creates Earth
Earth creates Metal
Metal holds Water
Water feeds Wood

The relationship must progress in this order. Only the Mother element can create the Child, in the same way that spring must follow winter. During moments of transition from one season to the next we can bring together a mix of practices inspired by the Mother element and the Child element for each of them to complement and strengthen the other. Here are some examples that show how to create the arc of a class using the Mother-Child relationship.

Winter to spring

INTENTION

- Acknowledge the ways that your ancestry contributes to your current strengths, and consider how this may lead to future possibilities.

- Cultivate kindness, vulnerability and humility.

- Set intentions and make plans.

- What wisdom will you carry with you into the future?

MOVEMENT

- Start in deep restorative postures emphasising twists and backbends.

- Gradually stir the body towards more energetic, rhythmic movements.

- Use circular motions on the ground, and then evolve to angular lines and standing balances.

- Shake, turn, jump, kick, reach, curl in and radiate outwards.

- Remember how the Bladder and Gallbladder meridians flow

downwards from the head to the feet, running along the back and outer seams of the legs. On the inner legs, work upwards to the groin and into the ribcage for the Kidney and Liver meridians. On the outer legs, work down the outer hips to the hamstrings and calf muscles.

- Engage the more subtle tendons and ligaments such as those in the wrists, ankles, hands and feet.

- Build stability from deep within, bringing awareness to the bones and skeletal structure.

Spring to early summer

INTENTION

- Cultivate friendliness and companionship.

- Explore the capacity for forgiveness.

- Encourage opportunities for creating community and for a greater sharing of individual riches.

- Revisit any unfulfilled ambition and consider giving it another try.

MOVEMENT

- Use energetic twists to generate heat.

- Establish rhythmic repetitions and maintain the pace in a way that is sustainable.

- At an appropriate moment, slow down to a simmering core sequence.

- Use heart-opening postures and poses that activate the chest muscles, obliques and inner arms.

- Open the voice for chanting.

- Where appropriate, use humour, laughter and music.

- Allow some time for self-practice or some partner work.

- Visualise the flow of energy from the heart to the fingers along the inside of the arms (Heart and Pericardium meridians) and from the fingers up the outside of the arms, over the shoulders and into the sides of the head (Small Intestine and Triple Heater meridians). Remind the students to observe the Liver and Gallbladder meridians up and down the legs and under the ribcage during lunges and twists.

Mid-summer to late summer

INTENTION

- Cultivate integrity in the flesh and in the spirit.

- Make space for whole-hearted presence in thought, word and deed.

- Encourage contentment, gratitude and acceptance of the present moment and of individual circumstances.

MOVEMENT

- Work at a steady pace, without rushing, without sudden changes.

- Provide variations and choices for all levels based on not only physical ability, but also the sheer joy of having multiple choices.

- Use core work to generate heat.

- Emphasise the connection to the ground.

- Bring awareness to the feet during transitions.

- Touch the ground with the hands and body.

- Use gravity as a prop.

- Use touch – either in the form of partner work or self-touch – to encourage sensitivity of the flesh and skin, as well as to build fuller proprioception.

- Draw attention to the centre of the palms, the *Lao Gong* point.

- Encourage students to move with their eyes closed where appropriate and safe.

- Emphasise the downward trajectory of the Stomach meridian and the upward climb of the Spleen meridian up the inner legs into the armpits.

- Move from standing, swirling poses to seated poses.

- Initiate movements that start away from the body and graduate towards the centre line of the body.

Late summer to autumn

INTENTION

- Shake off any excess extroversion of late summer.

- Acknowledge the beauty that has been, and leave the past behind.

- Identify what is of utmost value and do what is necessary to preserve and treasure it.

- Distil, condense, consolidate, trim, simplify.

- Be precise. Reduce the fluff. Be clean and clear, like the best-cut diamond in the world.

MOVEMENT

- Simplify. Go back to basics. Prioritise what is essential.

- Teach breathing practices that emphasise exhalation.

- Loosen the ribs and intercostal muscles to enable freer movement of the diaphragm.

- Emphasise internal and external rotation in the shoulders and arms to stimulate the Lung and Large Intestine meridians.

- Practise sinking into the legs and shake off weight from the upper body.

- Encourage meditation at the start or the end of the class with a clear and simple intention.

Autumn to winter

INTENTION

- Examine the perspective of time.

- Trust the unknown.

- Reflect, contemplate, journal.

MOVEMENT

- Practise long silent meditations after a period of strong breath exercise.

- Use forward folds and backbends to focus on the Kidney and Bladder meridians in active and restorative postures. Remember that healthy bodies of water must move, like the widest rivers and deepest oceans.

- Focus on building steadiness and integrity in the bones.

- Use inversions to address fear, the emotion most associated with the water element and our survival instinct.

- End classes with longer periods in Restorative or Yin Yoga poses.

- Consider including Yoga Nidra or a guided meditation during relaxation.

Part 3: Pairing meridians

As we move our limbs and trunk, all meridians naturally receive some degree of stimulation. What makes the difference is where we choose to focus and place our intention. Here are three ways to create meaningful pairings of meridians:

- Brothers and Sisters

- Six Levels of Energy

- Harmonising Dissonance.

Brothers and Sisters

The twelve meridians can be assigned a role as a 'Brother' or 'Sister' based on the *yin* or *yang* aspects of each meridian.

	Wood	Fire	Earth	Metal	Water
Sister (*yin*)	Liver	Heart, Pericardium	Spleen	Lung	Kidneys
Brother (*yang*)	Gallbladder	Small Intestine, Triple Heater	Stomach	Large Intestine	Bladder

When we work within one element, we stimulate both the Brother and Sister aspects of that element. When we combine two elements, as suggested in the seasonal transition sequences, we work on four meridians: the Brother-Sister pairs in both the Mother element and the Child elements.

Six Levels of Energy

A second way to pair meridians is to use the Six Levels of Energy, a classification system in Chinese medicine. These levels are morphological and are used to identify which meridians require acupuncture treatment, according to where symptoms of disease are present in the patient. These six levels are also called the Three Yin and Three Yang, and are sometimes used as a basis for explaining the principles of *yin* and *yang*. The diagrams below illustrate how they are expressed on the body. Movements that are directed at each of these anatomical areas will stimulate the corresponding pairs of meridians.

The following diagrams show the locations of the Three Yang and Three Yin.

Yang Ming (Bright Yang) is indicated on the figure on the left. These areas on the side of the head, along the arms and down the front of the body correspond to the meridians of the Large Intestine and the Stomach.

Shao Yang (Lesser Yang) is indicated on the figure in the middle. These areas on the side of the head, the lateral seam of the arms, the torso and the legs correspond to the meridians of the Triple Heater and the Gallbladder.

Tai Yang (Great Yang) is indicated on the figure on the right. These areas on the head, the back of the arms, shoulders, down the spine and legs correspond to the meridians of the Small Intestine and the Bladder. The area in the middle of the head in the figure on the left is also *Tai Yang*.

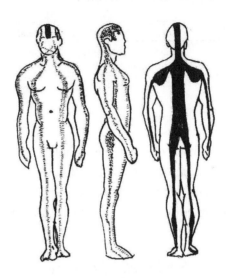

The Three Yin pairs are the Lung and the Spleen, called *Tai Yin* (Great Yin); the Kidneys and the Heart, called *Shao Yin* (Lesser Yin); the Pericardium and the Liver, called *Jue Yin* (Extreme Yin).

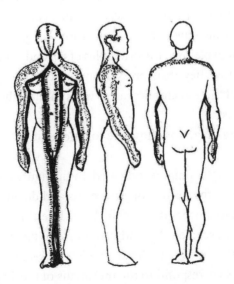

The *yin* meridians and corresponding areas are concentrated on the front of the body, the inner seams of the legs and along the arms. The darkened area on the figure on the left indicates the *Shao Yin* (Lesser Yin). This area corresponds to the Heart meridian and the Kidney meridian. On the medial side of the Kidney meridian is the Liver meridian. On the lateral side of the Kidney meridian is the Spleen meridian. The Pericardium and Lung meridians run along the arms.

Harmonising Dissonance

Imbalances in the functioning of organ systems lead to disease. These imbalances could be in the relationship between the Five Elements. Within this framework, when imbalances occur, one solution is to adjust the Mother-Child relationship. The other option is to call in the Grandmother. Here is a reminder of how this relationship of respect and restraint works:

Grandmother and Grandchild
Fire melts Metal
Metal chops Wood
Wood covers Earth
Earth dams Water
Water douses Fire

To bring harmony, we engage only the *yin* organ meridian to rebalance the body. Combine the meridian-specific practices provided in Chapter 4 with other postures and movements to invigorate and sooth the imbalance you are seeking to harmonise.

HARMONISING FIRE AND METAL: HEART AND LUNG

Imbalances occur when there is either excess or deficiency in one or both elements. This could be expressed as excessive grief, obsessive minimalism, harshness, solitude, depression or coldness.

Perform exercises to stimulate the Heart and Lung meridians to smooth, soothe and cool any friction, or to warm, loosen or lubricate what is stuck or hardened. When sufficiently warmed, metal becomes pliable, allowing magnificent transformations to occur. Consider themes related to matters of the heart, forgiveness and intellectual or spiritual inspiration.

HARMONISING METAL AND WOOD: LUNG AND LIVER

Imbalances in this relationship occur when purity is lost, or when toxicity overburdens the system and the liver and lungs fail to function well. When we are overburdened, initiating any action becomes more difficult, and hope is progressively lost.

Perform exercises to stimulate the Lung and Liver meridians, to decongest, detoxify, cool, rehydrate and dislodge any stagnation. Figuratively cut through the mess, clear out the rubbish, re-establish the virtuous path and take the necessary steps towards any unfulfilled ambitions and dreams.

HARMONISING WOOD AND EARTH: LIVER AND SPLEEN

When weighed down by overthinking or over-planning, overburdened and overwhelmed by having taken on too much, the Liver and Spleen can start to sag under pressure. This can be expressed as lethargy, panic, inability to make wise choices or the inability to start or complete a task.

Perform exercises to stimulate elimination, promote circulation and improve digestion. Encourage practices that will unblock the flow of what naturally needs to be released, such as sweat or tears. Encourage practices that provide clarity of thought and straightforward action.

HARMONISING EARTH AND WATER: SPLEEN AND KIDNEYS

When hydration is not appropriately supplied and distributed, everything suffers. The body reacts with inflammation of the joints, swelling, stiffness, puffiness in the extremities, dry skin, dry eyes, diarrhoea and urination difficulties. Soil that is baked dry cannot hold any water. Water simply runs off the surface. Inversely, when soil is sodden, it cannot hold its form.

Perform exercises to promote stability, using a regular rhythm. Encourage wise and mature decision-making. Use movements to promote flow and the release of excessive heaviness.

HARMONISING WATER AND FIRE: KIDNEY AND HEART

When water and fire come into contact, there is the fizz of an alchemical reaction. These are the ingredients that make life. Many traditions recognise the magic that happens when water and fire meet. An imbalance in these two elements comes across simply as the absence of magic: a lacklustre existence, an absence of zing. The person is disheartened, unenthusiastic, unable to see or appreciate the wonder and magic that surround every life. This imbalance can also manifest as manic behaviour, swinging from euphoria to extreme fatigue. The heart is not well and the essences required to fuel life are stressed.

Encourage practices of self-care. Encourage a reconnection to family and community spirit. Allow plenty of rest, and focus on replenishing the kidneys and warming the heart.

Part 4: Inspiration from Chinese herbalism

Chinese herbs are categorised by their properties based on several measures: being relatively *yin* (cool, cold) or relatively *yang* (warm, hot), their taste (sour, salty, bitter, sweet, acrid, pungent or spicy), their colour and their shape, and the effect they have on the qi.

Our qi is likely to react in one of the following four ways when the correct medicinal herbs are used to treat a symptom:

- Strengthen that which is weak.

- Condense that which is light.

- Move that which is stagnant.

- Expel that which is toxic.

These four qualities can be used as a foundation for designing a suitable sequence, layered with influences and other themes from the Five Elements.

Strengthen

- Replenish and enliven that which is depleted or empty.

- Rejuvenate that which is tired.

- Nourish the weak and distressed.

- Beyond learning a skill, become competent in it.

- Amplify what is good, wise and skilful.

- Enhance what is already progressing well.

- Raise self-esteem.

- Renew intentions and ambitions.

- Provide substance to ideas and plans.

Condense

- Gather in, consolidate, concentrate, tighten and secure. Add tonicity, such as through isometric movements.

- Stop leakage or accidental loss. Retain what is vital and useful.

- Reunite that which has been stretched to excess.

- Regulate intensity, gravity or density, lightening or saturating as necessary.

- Prioritise and preserve that which is essential.

- Feed, enrich, intensify, bolster, deepen, sweeten that which we inherently know is good for us.

Move

- Circulate with greater vigour that which is sluggish or stagnant.

- Distribute or redistribute any excesses to promote cohesion and evenness.

- Disperse that which is pooled, congealed, clogged, cornered or stuck.

- Promote flow, fluidity and radiance.

- Relax, loosen, liberate and lubricate tightness in body, breath and mind.

- Regulate slackness, administer a rhythm, establish a schedule, modulate the tempo.

- Shake off and free up. Fizz, like Champagne bubbles.

- Change perspectives, locations and views.

- Refresh tired habits.

Expel

- Sweat out, exhale, purge or evacuate toxins and excess fluid.

- Dump the rubbish – figuratively and physically.

- Dismantle or remove mental barriers.

- Cleanse and refresh that which has been neglected.

- Forgive.

- Drop the old baggage. Stop repeating destructive habits.

- Find closure.

POSTSCRIPT

Integration

In the following passage, from Chapter 25 of the *Tao Te Ching*, humanity is placed on an equal plane to the Tao, the universe and the earth:

> The Tao is great.
> The universe is great.
> Earth is great.
> Man is great.
> These are the four great powers.[1]

The word used to mean great is *da*, which means big, large, mature, elder or wise. The spirit within us that identifies as 'I' or 'me' is seen as divine, magical, mysterious and great. The tissue, blood and bones that bind together to make our body carry the same wonder contained in the stars, the trees, the minerals, the largest animals, the smallest microbes, sunshine and serendipity.

Every effort to improve our selves contributes to making life better for all. We are woven into the fabric of the universe as it pulses – contracting and expanding. Within the microcosm of our physical bodies, our lives and our minds, we are part of a rhythm and flow that is greater than conscious thought, ego or worldly concerns. When we engage with life in all its expressions, when

---

1   Mitchell, S. (1988) *Tao Te Ching: A New English Version*. New York: Harper & Row

we do the things that fill rather than deplete us, we make life better for the earth, the universe and the Dao.

We will never know everything, and yet we generally know more than we think we do. The knowledge in this book is for you to play with, adapt and develop so that you can use it to improve more lives.

'Energy flows where attention goes' is a phrase often quoted by teachers of qigong. By training our mind to direct the flow of qi, we create strength. The strength available depends on the quality of qi that is being cultivated, which in turn depends on the intentions that you sow. My intention is for you to explore how you cultivate qi and how you experience the meridians and the Five Elements, and to trust the choices that you make on your journey.

GLOSSARY OF CHINESE TERMS AND PRONUNCIATION GUIDE

All Chinese terms are presented below in Hanyu Pinyin alongside traditional Chinese characters, listed in the order that they appear in the book. Barring a few exceptions, I have used English words to approximate the pronunciation of each word. For brevity, the pronunciation guide is provided only once in the first appearance of the word.

Chapter 1

Jing 精: Vital essence, sexual fluids. Pronounced *ching*.

Qi 氣: Energy, breath, life force. Pronounced *chee* like in *cheek*.

Shen 神: Spirit, god, divinity. Pronounced *sh-urn* like in *burn*.

Yi Jin Jing 易筋經: The earliest known text of the *Yi Jin Jing* dates to the early 19th century. However, the contents of the *Muscle/Tendon Change Classic* are believed to date back as far as the Liang Dynasty (502 CE) and are believed to have originated in a Shaolin monastery. The *Yi Jin Jing* is known for 12 exercises, each corresponding to a meridian. Here, *yi* (pronounced *yee*) means to change, *jin* (pronounced like *chin*) means tendons or muscles and *jing* (pronounced *ching*) means method.

Hun 魂: Pronounced *hwen*, the *hun* is a type of soul in Chinese philosophy. Associated with the Wood element, the *hun* detaches from the body after death. It contains the components *yun* 云 (pronounced like *Ewan*) meaning cloud, and *gui* 鬼 (pronounced *gway*) meaning ghost. The *hun* is sometimes called the immortal soul.

Po 魄: The *po* (pronounced *pw-or*) is the mortal soul that stays attached to the body after death. The character is also drawn with *gui* 鬼 (ghost) but contains the character for *bai* 白 (pronounced *buy*), which usually means white but also means plain or empty. The *po* is associated with the Metal element.

Yong yi, bu yong li 用意, 不用力: Use intention, do not use force. The *-o* in *Yong* is pronounced like in *oh*. It means to use. *Yi* is pronounced like *he* and means intention. *Bu* (pronounced *boo*) means no. *Li* (pronounced *lee*) means strength.

You yi, you qi, you li 有意, 有氣, 有力: This literally means have intention, have energy, have strength. Within the context of qigong, the phrase means 'When we practise, we start with our intention.' The intention comes before the qi (here meaning breath or energy) which in turn comes before strength or power. This phrase captures how qigong encourages physical restraint and moderation in expending physical strength, favouring intention and breath over muscularity. The *-ou* in *you* is pronounced like *owe*. It means to have or to exist.

Yi 意: Intention. The character is composed of the character for sound, 音 *yin*, and the character for heart, 心 *xin*. The character for sound is made up of the characters 立 *li*, and 日 *ri*.

Li 立: To stand, to be vertical, be upright. Pronounced *lee*.

Ri 日: The sun. Also means date or day. Pronounced *rr*.

Xin 心: The heart. Pronounced *sin*. The character is also used to compose words relating to emotions and thoughts such as love, anger, fear, kindness, grace, ambition, to read, to think, to miss someone, to believe, to neglect, to be steady.

Gong 功: Merit or achievement. The *g* in *gong* is pronounced like in *gould*, the *-ong* is pronounced *-oong*.

Qigong 氣功: This Chinese system of physical exercises, massage, breathing techniques and meditation for cultivating energy dates back thousands of years. Very few ancient texts exist on the subject, and the tradition is still mostly transmitted orally. In the mid-20th century, the Chinese government attempted to standardise the practice. One of the results was the mass popularisation of the practice in China. Today, thousands of disparate practices use the term qigong. Consistent throughout these different lineages are practices to regulate the body, *tiao shen* 調身, to regulate the breath, *tiao xi* 調息, and to regulate the mind, *tiao xin* 調心.

Chapter 2

Huxi 呼吸: Breath, breathing, pronounced *hoo-see.*

Xiqi 吸氣: Inhalation, pronounced *see-chee.* The use of the word qi indicates that the inhalation is the intake of energy.

Huqi 呼氣: Exhalation, pronounced *hoo-chee.*

Ma shang lai! 馬上來: Right away, it's on the way. Literally translates as horse, on, coming. The *-a* in *ma* is pronounced like in the sound *baa*, *-ang* in *shang* is like *hung*, *lai* is like *lie.*

Kuo 擴: To expand. Also used to mean extend, enlarge or spread. The *k* is pronounced like *kh-* in *khan.* The *-uo* is pronounced like *war.*

Suo 縮: To shrink. Also used to mean reduce, contract or withdraw. Pronounced like *swore.*

Man 滿: Full. Also used as a verb to mean to fill or fulfil. As an adjective it can also mean satisfied or fully packed. The *-an* is pronounced like in the name *Sîan* or *Oman.*

Kong 空: Empty. Also means sky, air or in vain. The *ko-* is pronounced like in *coat.*

Que 缺: Lack, absence or a vacancy. The *q* is pronounced *ch* like in *chin.* The *-ue* is pronounced *wear.*

Qi 起: To rise, to initiate, to start. Pronounced *chee.* The tone of the *-i* is pronounced like when asking *please?*

Yi qi 一起: together. Pronounced *ee-chee.*

Dui bu qi 對不起: I am sorry. Pronounced *dway-boo-chee.*

Chen 沉: To sink, to submerge, to drop. As an adjective, it also means profound, deep, heavy. Pronounced like *churn.*

Chen jing 沉靜: Peaceful, calm, quiet. *Jing* pronounced *chin.*

Chen si 沉思: Contemplation or meditation. *Si* pronounced like *sci-* in *scissors.*

Chen ji 沉寂: Silence or stillness. *Ji* pronounced *chee* like in *cheese.*

Chen zhuo 沉著: Steady, calm and collected. *Zh* pronounced *ch-*, *-uo* pronounced *war.*

Chen jin 沉浸: To immerse or to soak in. *Jin* pronounced *chin.*

Chen mi 沉迷: Deeply engrossed, addicted. *Mi* pronounced *mee.*

Chen men 沉悶: Oppressive (of weather), depressed. *-men* is pronounced like in *women.*

Chen zhong 沉重: Harsh and critical. *Zhong* pronounced *jong,* with *jo-* like in *joe.*

Chen mo 沉默: Uncommunicative. *Mo* pronounced *more.*

Kuai ma jia bian 快馬加鞭: To spur on a swift horse. *Kuai,* meaning fast, pronounced *k-why. Ma,* horse. *Jia,* to add, pronounced *chee-ah. Bian,* whip, pronounced *bee-anne.*

Jia su 加速: Increase velocity, accelerate. *Su,* velocity, pronounced like *sue.*

Ning jing zhi yuan 寧靜致遠: Enduring accomplishments are achieved by leading a quiet life. *Ning,* meaning peaceful. *Jing,* meaning stillness, pronounced *ching. Zhi,* meaning to deliver, pronounced *chrr* like in *chirp. Yuan,* meaning far, pronounced *you-anne.*

Jian su 減速: Reduce velocity, decelerate. *Jian* pronounced *chee-anne.*

Ruo 弱: Absence of resistance, weakness, vulnerability. Pronounced like *raw.*

Feng Shui 風水: *Feng* is wind and *shui* is water. *Feng Shui* is a system of laws concerning the orientation of a building, the use of a space or the placement of furniture to bring harmony and prosperity. *Feng Shui* principles are devised using a combination of the directions of a compass, the *bagua* 八卦 (also called the Eight Trigrams), the Five Elements and the Chinese zodiac. *Fe-* in *Feng* is pronounced like in *fur. Shui* is pronounced *sh-way.*

Zhi nan zhen 指南針: A compass. Literally, point south needle. *Zhi* pronounced *chrr, nan* like in *Sîan, zhen* like *churn.*

Fan zhe 反者: A rebound, a return, a contrary movement. Famously used in the *Dao De Jing* Chapter 40 by Lao Tzu: 反者道之动. 弱者道之用. *Fan zhe dao zhi dong. Ruo zhe dao zhi yong.* A rebound is the way the Dao moves. Absence of resistance is how the Dao is used. The *-an* of *fan* is pronounced like in the name *Sîan. Zhe* is pronounced *chur* like in *church.*

Wai dan gong 外丹功: External martial arts, where energy is directed from the outer limbs inwards. This practice includes the use of herbal medicines and minerals. *Wai* pronounced like in *wide. Dan* pronounced like in *Sîan,* here meaning alchemy. The same word *dan* is used for *dantian,* the centres of energy on the body.

Nei dan gong 内丹功: Internal martial arts, where energy is directed from the centre of the body towards the outer limbs. *Nei* like in *neighbour. Wai dan gong* and *nei dan gong* are Daoist practices for the body, mind and spirit to promote longevity of body and spirit.

Wai zhuang 外壯: Physical strength and stability resulting from qigong practice. *Zhu* in *zhuang* pronounced *choo, -ang* like in *lung*.

Nei zhuang 內壯: Strength in the form of a stable mind, a vibrant spirit and enduring willpower resulting from qigong practice.

Chapter 3

Yin 陰: The shady side of the mountain. The following qualities are often regarded as *yin*: cool, female, dense, deep, passive, wet, hidden, descending, the moon, space.

Yang 陽: The sunny side of the mountain. The following qualities are often regarded as *yang*: warm, male, open, active, dry, rising, hollow, expansion, the sun, time. The pronunciation of *-ang* is as in *young*, and not like in *hang*.

Hui Yin 會陰: Meeting of the Yin. Acupuncture point on the perineum, also called Ren-1 or CV1. *Hui* pronounced *h-way*.

Yao Yang Guan 腰陽關: Gateway to the Yang Energy of the Loins. Acupuncture point on the Governor Vessel located between the fourth and fifth lumbar vertebrae, also called Du-3 or GV3. *Yao* pronounced like *yow-* in *yowl*. *Guan* is *kw-one*.

Ming Men 命門: Gateway of Life. Acupuncture point on the Governor Vessel located between the second and third lumbar vertebrae, also called Du-4 or GV4. *Men* pronounced as in *women*.

Zhong Shu 中樞: Central or Middle Pivot. Acupuncture point on the Governor Vessel located between the seventh and eighth thoracic vertebrae, also called Du-7 or GV7. *Zhong* pronounced *ch-oh-ng. Shu* like *shoe*.

Ling Tai 靈臺: Elevated Platform or Tower for the Spirit. Acupuncture point on the Governor Vessel located between sixth and seventh thoracic vertebrae, also called Du-10 or GV10. *Tai* like in *Thailand*.

Shen Dao 神道: The Pathway of the Spirit. Acupuncture point on the Governor Vessel located between the fifth and sixth vertebrae, also called Du-11 or GV11.

Da Zhui 大椎: Great Hammer. Acupuncture point on the Governor Vessel located between the seventh cervical and the first thoracic vertebrae, also called Du-14 or GV14. *Zhui* pronounced *chew-way*.

Feng Fu 風府: Wind Palace. Acupuncture point on the Governor Vessel located at the base of the occiput, also called Du-16 or GV16. The *-e* in *feng* is pronounced like in *shirt*. *Fu* pronounced *foo*.

Bai Hui 百會: One Hundred Meetings. Acupuncture point on the Governor Vessel located at the top of the skull, also called Du-20 or GV20. *Bai* pronounced like *buy*. *Hui* pronounced *h-way*.

Yin Tang 印堂: Hall of Impressions. This acupuncture point is located on the forehead between the eyebrows. It is considered an extraordinary point and does not follow the conventional numbered naming system. *Tang* pronounced like *hung*.

Dantian 丹田: Cinnabar field. There are three points on the body that are considered centres of energy, called *dantian*. The upper *dantian* is on the forehead, near *Yin Tang*, the middle *dantian* is at the level of the heart and the lower *dantian* is in the lower belly, approximately three fingers below the navel. *Dan* pronounced *tah-n*. *Tian* pronounced *tee-anne*.

Cheng Jiang 承漿: Receiving of Broth (Fluid). Acupuncture point on the Conception Vessel located in the dip just below the lower lip, also called Ren-24 or CV24. *Cheng* pronounced like *churn*. *Jiang* pronounced *chee-ung*.

Lian Quan 廉泉: Angled or Crooked Spring. Acupuncture point on the Conception Vessel located on the throat below the hyoid bone, also called Ren-23 or CV23. *Lian* pronounced *lee-anne*, *quan* pronounced *chew-anne*.

Tian Tu 天突: Heaven Rushes Out. Acupuncture point on the Conception Vessel located on the throat below the cricoid cartilage, also called Ren-22 or CV22. *Tian* pronounced *tea-yen*, *tu* like *too*.

Yu Tang 玉堂: Jade Hall or Court. Acupuncture point on the Conception Vessel located at the level of the third intercostal space, also called Ren-18 or CV18. *Yu* pronounced like in *pew* or *queue*.

Zi Gong 紫宮: Purple Palace. Acupuncture point on the Conception Vessel located at the level of the second intercostal space, also called Ren-19 or CV19. *Zi* pronounced *t'zeuh*. The *g* in *gong* is like in *gould*. The *-o* in *gong* is pronounced *oh*.

Xuan Ji 璇璣: Jade and Irregular Pearl. Acupuncture point on the Conception Vessel located in the notch between the collarbones, at the base of the throat. Also called Ren-21 or CV21. *Xuan* pronounced like *sue-anne*. *Ji* pronounced *chee*.

Shen Que 神闕: Watchtower of the Spirit. Acupuncture point on the Conception

Vessel located in the navel. Also called Ren-8 or CV8. *Que* pronounced *chew-air*.

Ju Que 巨闕: Gateway to the Imperial City. Acupuncture point on the Conception Vessel located at the level of the epigastrium, where the thorax meets the abdomen, about two fingers below the xiphoid process. Also called Ren-14 or CV14. *Ju* pronounced like *chew*.

Shang Wan 上脘: Upper Cavity or Duct. Acupuncture point on the Conception Vessel on the abdomen located about two fingers below CV14. Also called Ren-13 or CV13. *Shang* pronounced *sh-hung*. *Wan* like *one*.

Zhong Wan 中脘: Middle Cavity or Duct. Acupuncture point on the Conception Vessel on the abdomen located about two fingers below CV13. Also called Ren-12 or CV12.

Xia Wan 下脘: Lower Cavity or Duct. Acupuncture point on the Conception Vessel about four fingers above the navel. Also called Ren-10 or CV10. *Xia* pronounced *see-ah*.

Shi Men 石門: Stone Gateway. Acupuncture point on the Conception Vessel about a hand's width below the navel. Also called Ren-5 or CV5. *Shi* pronounced *shrr*. *Men* like in *women*.

Guan Yuan 關元: First or Original Mountain Pass. Acupuncture point on the Conception Vessel about four fingers above the pubic symphysis. Also called Ren-4 or CV4. *Yuan* pronounced *you-anne*.

Shibashi 十八式: Eighteen forms. A sequence of movements developed by Lin Housheng 林厚省 in 1979 in Shanghai. It has since been popularised and used around the world as a practice in itself and as a warm up for various martial arts practices. There are eight *Shibashi* sequences, each containing a sequence of 18 movements. *Shi* is pronounced *shrr*. *Ba* is *baa*.

Yong Quan 涌泉: Bubbling Spring. Acupuncture point on the Kidney meridian located on the sole of the foot between the second and third metatarsal bones. Also called Ki-1. *Yong* like in *yo-yo*.

Lao Gong 勞宮: Palace of Toil or Weariness. Acupuncture point on the Pericardium meridian located on the palm of the hand between the fourth and fifth metacarpals. Also called PC-8. *Lao* pronounced like in *loud*, *gong* pronounced *koong*.

Tian Chong 天衝: With the Full Force of Heaven. Acupuncture point on the Gallbladder meridian located on the side of the head above the ear. Also called GB-9. The *-o* in *chong* is pronounced *oh*.

Wei Dao 維道: Binding Path. Acupuncture point on the Gallbladder meridian located on the hip, also called GB-28. *Wei* like *way*.

Zheng Ying 正營: A Correct or Upright Way of Being. Acupuncture point on the Gallbladder meridian located on top of the skull, about a finger's width away from the midline, approximately in line with the top of the earlobe. Also called GB-17. *Zheng* pronounced *churn-ng*.

Ri Yue 日月: Sun and Moon. Acupuncture point on the Gallbladder meridian located in the seventh intercostal space, directly under the nipple. Also called GB-24. *Ri* pronounced *rr*. *Yue* pronounced *you-air*.

Guang Ming 光明: Bright and Clear. Acupuncture point on the Gallbladder meridian located on the front edge of the fibula, approximately a quarter of the way up from the ankle towards the knee crease. Also called GB-37. *Guang* pronounced *kw-ung*.

Yang Ling Quan 陽陵泉: Spring of Yang Energy. Acupuncture point on the Gallbladder meridian located just below the knee, on the lower forward corner of the head of the fibula. Also called GB-34.

Qiu Xu 丘墟: A Mound in the Wilderness. Acupuncture point on the Gallbladder meridian located under the extensor digitorum longus tendon where it goes over the fourth metatarsal of the foot at the ankle joint. Also called GB-40. *Qiu* pronounced *chee-oh*. *Xu* pronounced like *sui-* in *suit*.

Da Dun 大敦: Great Honesty or Esteem. Acupuncture point on the Liver meridian located on the lateral edge of the big toe. Also called Liv-1. *Dun* pronounced *two-urn*.

Qi Men 期門: Gateway of Expectations and Hope. Acupuncture point on the Liver meridian. Some schools locate this point in the sixth intercostal space directly under the nipple, while some schools locate this point on the nipple line but on the bottom edge of the ribcage. Also known as Liv-14. *Qi* pronounced *chee*.

Yun Men 雲門: Gateway of Clouds. Acupuncture point on the Lung meridian located in the dip under the end of the collarbone. Also called Lu-2. *Yun* pronounced *you-win*.

Tian Fu 天府: Celestial or Heavenly Palace. Acupuncture point on the Lung meridian located on the upper arm along the outer border of the bicep muscles approximately a third of the way down from the armpit to the elbow crease. Also called Lu-3. *Fu* pronounced *foo*.

Xia Bai 俠白: Valiant or Heroic White. Acupuncture point on the Lung meridian located approximately a finger's distance below Lu-3. Also called Lu-4. *Xia* pronounced *see-ah. Bai* like *buy*.

He Gu 合谷: A Union of Valleys. Acupuncture point on the Large Intestine meridian located on the back of the hand, in the angle where the thumb and index finger meet. Also called LI-4. *He* pronounced *her*. The *g-* in *gu* is pronounced like in *gould; -u* is pronounced as *-oo*.

Xue Hai 血海: Sea of Blood. Acupuncture point located on the Spleen meridian on the medial surface of the thigh approximately four fingers above the knee. Also called SP-10. *Xue* pronounced *sh-wear. Hai* like *high*.

Chapter 4

Fang Song Gong 放鬆功: Active relaxation taught in certain schools of qigong. The premise of the practice is that the pathways for qi open when the mind, breath and body are relaxed. With practice, one can learn to find comfort and relax the entire body, including the internal organs, while in any physical position. *Fang song* means relaxation. *Fang* is pronounced *far-ng. Song* is pronounced *soong*.

Shen Shu 腎俞: Access Point to the Kidneys. Acupuncture point on the Bladder meridian located on the back approximately three fingers away from the middle of the spine, at the level between the second and third lumbar vertebrae. Also called BL-23. *Shen* pronounced *sh-urn. Shu* like *shoe*.

Qi Hai Shu 氣海俞: Access Point to a Sea of Qi. Acupuncture point on the Bladder meridian located at the level between the third and fourth lumbar vertebrae below BL-23. Also called BL-24.

Huang Men 肓門: Gateway of Vitality. Acupuncture on the Bladder meridian located on the level between the first and second lumbar vertebrae about a hand's distance from the middle of the spine. Also called BL-46 or 51. *Huang* pronounced *who-arng*.

Zhi Shi 志室: Residence of the Will or Hall of Ambition. Acupuncture point on the Bladder meridian located two fingers below BL-46. Also called BL-47 or 52. Note the presence of the character for heart, *xin 心*, in the composition of the character for *zhi*, meaning will or willpower. *Zhi* pronounced *chrr. Shi* pronounced *shrr*.

Tian Liao 天髎: Heavenly Bone. Acupuncture point on the Triple Heater meridian located on the surface of the shoulder approximately in line with the upper tip of the scapula. Also called TH-15. *Li-* pronounced *lee*. *-ao* pronounced like *ow-* in *owl*.

Tian You 天牖: Heavenly Window. Acupuncture point on the Triple Heater meridian located below the mastoid bone, forward of the sternocleidomastoid, under the earlobe. Also called TH-16. *You* pronounced *yee-owe*.

Qu Quan 曲泉: Crooked Spring. Acupuncture point on the Liver meridian located on the inner leg at the knee crease. Also called Liv-8. *Qu* pronounced *ch-wee*. *Quan* pronounced *ch-when*.

Zhang Wo 掌握: To hold the hand in a fist, to grasp, to master, to hold in one's hand, to wield. *Zhang* pronounced *ch-arng*. *Wo* like *war*.

Luohan Qigong 羅漢氣功: Also known as *Luohan Quan* 羅漢拳. This martial art has its roots in the Shaolin temple and Shaolin Kungfu tradition, one of the oldest styles of kungfu. It combines Buddhist philosophy and martial arts, and originated in Henan province in China. *Luohan* is the Chinese name for the Sanskrit equivalent *Arhat*, meaning one who is enlightened. *Luo* pronounced *loo-ore*. *Han* pronounced *harn*.

Hua Rou Men 滑肉門: Gateway of Food Lubrication. Acupuncture point on the Stomach meridian located approximately four fingers away from the middle of the navel and two fingers up. Also called ST-24. *Hua* pronounced *hoo-are*, *rou* like *row*.

Ru Zhong 乳中: Centre of the Breast. Acupuncture point on the Stomach meridian located in the middle of the nipple. Also called ST-17. *Ru* pronounced *roo*.

Chapter 5

Xing Yi Quan 興義拳: Fist of righteous intent. Although the history of this Chinese martial art is much disputed, *Xing Yi Quan* forms include the popular training methods of *Zhan Zhuang*, *Wuxing* (Five Element forms), *Shi Er Xing* (Twelve Animal Frolics) and movements with weapons such as the sabre, sword and spear. It is regarded as a style of internal martial arts.

Yu 魚: Fish, a symbol of wealth, abundance and prosperity. Pronounced *ywee*.

Yu 玉: Jade, prized for its durability and beauty. Also pronounced *ywee*.

Zhan Zhuang 站樁: Standing like a post. A standing form of qigong practice where postures are held for extended periods of time. The premise is that, with practice, the qi channels open while holding these postures. Beginners start by holding a posture for two to three minutes, with the aim of advancing to considerably longer periods. *Zhan* pronounced *ch-arn*. *Zhuang* pronounced *chw-arng*. See also *Xing Yi Quan*.

Chapter 6

Wuxing 五行: Five Ways or Elements. *Wu* pronounced *woo*. *Xing* pronounced *sing*. Also called the Five Movements, Five Phases or Five Stages. The Five Elements are *jin* 金 Metal, *mu* 木 Wood, *shui* 水 Water, *huo* 火 Fire and *tu* 土 Earth. The five are linked in a mutually generative relationship and a mutually controlling relationship. This system is found in many fields of Chinese philosophy and creativity including *Feng Shui*, martial arts, divination, Traditional Chinese Medicine, astrology, painting, cooking and music. *Jin* is pronounced like *chin*. *Mu* is like *moo*. *Shui* is pronounced *sh-way*. *Huo* is pronounced *who-or*. *Tu* is like *two*.

Yang Ming 陽明: Bright Yang. Corresponds to the Large Intestine and Stomach meridians.

Shao Yang 少陽: Lesser Yang. Corresponds to the Triple Heater and Gallbladder meridians. *-ao* in *shao* is like *how*.

Tai Yang 太陽: Great Yang. Corresponds to the Small Intestine and the Bladder meridians. *Tai* like in *Taiwan*.

Tai Yin 太陰: Great Yin. Corresponds to the Lung and Spleen meridians.

Shao Yin 少陰: Lesser Yin. Corresponds to the Kidney and Heart meridians.

Jue Yin 厥陰: Extreme or Faintest Yin. *Jue* pronounced *ch-wear*. Corresponds to the Pericardium and Liver meridians.

FURTHER STUDY

I trust and wholeheartedly recommend the following resources.

Teachers
Cameron Tukapua
Judith Hanson Lasater
Matthew Raymond Cohen
Mimi Kuo-Deemer
Max Strom
Donna Farhi
Sarah Powers
Gerad Kite
Elisabeth Rochat de la Vallée

Books on physical movement, yoga and qigong
Relax and Renew: Restful Yoga for Stressful Times. Judith Hanson Lasater, 1995
Teaching Yoga. Donna Farhi, 2006
Insight Yoga. Sarah Powers, 2008
A Life Worth Breathing. Max Strom, 2010
Walk Yourself Well. Sherry Brourman, 1998
Yoga Nidra. Richard Miller, 2005
Taking Root to Fly. Irene Dowd, 1981
Qigong and the Tai Chi Axis. Mimi Kuo-Deemer, 2018
The Way of Qigong: The Art and Science of Chinese Energy Healing. Kenneth S. Cohen, 1997
Qigong: The Secret of Youth. Dr Yang Jwing-Ming, 2000
Baguazhang: Theory and Applications. Master Liang Shou-Yu and Dr Yang Jwing-Ming, 2008
The Root of Chinese Chi Kung. Dr Yang Jwing-Ming, 1989
The Way of Energy. Master Lam Kam Chuen, 1991

Books on Chinese medicine and acupuncture
The Five Elements in Classical Chinese Text. Elisabeth Rochat de la Vallée, 2009
A Study of Qi. Elisabeth Rochat de la Vallée, 2006
The Heart. Claude Larre and Elisabeth Rochat de la Vallée, 1991

Characters of Wisdom: Taoist Tales of the Acupuncture Points. Debra Kaatz, 2005
Classical Five-Element Acupuncture Volume 3. Prof JR Worsley
Between Heaven and Earth: A Guide to Chinese Medicine. Harriet Beinfield and Efrem Korngold
Opening Up: A Conversation About How to be Real. Cameron Tukapua, 2013

Appreciating life, nature and each of the Five Elements

Tao Te Ching: A New English Version. Lao Tzu translated by Stephen Mitchell, 1988
The World's Religions. Huston Smith, 1991
Living Beautifully with Uncertainty and Change. Pema Chodron, 2012
Bird by Bird. Anne Lamott, 1995
The Architecture and Design of Man and Woman. Alexander Tsiaras and Barry Werth, 2004
Tattoos on the Heart. Gregory Boyle, 2010
Messages from Water. Masaro Emoto, 1999
Divine Beauty. John O'Donohue, 2003
Benedictus. John O'Donohue, 2007
Life on Earth. David Attenborough, 2018
Wilding: The Return of Nature to a British Farm. Isabella Tree, 2019
From Bacteria to Bach and Back: The Evolution of Minds. Daniel C. Dennett
Wild Flowers of Britain and Ireland. Marjorie Blamey, Richard Fitter and Alastair Fitter, 2003
Trees of Britain and Northern Europe. David More and John White, 2003
Wild Animals of Britain and Europe. Nicholas Arnold, Denys Ovenden and Gordon Corbet, 1994
The Concise Guide to Self-Sufficiency. John Seymour, 2007
The Seven Basic Plots. Christopher Booker, 2004
The 5 Love Languages. Gary Chapman, 1992
Salt, Fat, Acid, Heat. Samin Nosrat, 2017
Waiting For Godot. Samuel Beckett, 1952

SUBJECT INDEX

abundance 44, 102, 122, 147
accelerate 32, 36, 141
acupuncture 14, 38, 41, 54, 129
air, in emptiness 34
amenorrhea 54
ancestry 37, 118, 124
anchor, point in a posture 30, 37–8, 48, 86,
    94, 123
arms
    bringing qi to 97
    in sequencing 115, 121, 125, 126, 129–131
apnoea 29
asthma 29
autumn 114, 127–8

bamboo 22–3
back, as in dorsal
    in Horse Stance 31
    meridians on 40, 45, 49, 50
    see also bladder meridian; kidney
        meridian
backbends 89, 121, 124, 128
bladder meridian 50, 63–5, 119
blockage 49, 54, 76
blood 120
blood circulation, blood flow 18, 23, 30, 38,
    56, 97
blood clots 54
blood, disorders 54
blood pulse 18
blood vessels 120

body hair 114
bone 118
bone marrow 118
breath, breathing 21, 28–30, 39, 41
breath, retention
breathing exercises 41–5, 88–91
breathing conditions 29
breath, regulating the 28

central axis 46, 48
central meridians 40, 41
centre 37, 123, 126–7
cervical spine 42
chanting 114, 125
chaos 24, 43, 120
chronic obstructive pulmonary disease 29
clavicle 50, 52–3
coccyx see tailbone
Conception Vessel 40–3, 50, 68, 69
contentment 20, 34, 126
control issues 53
cool, cooling 24, 72, 89, 118, 119, 131, 132,
    133
cystic fibrosis 29

Dao De Jing see Mitchell, S.
decelerate 32, 37, 141
deep channels 48, 55
density 33, 36, 44, 134
depression 64, 131

diaphragm 42, 50, 52, 68, 89, 115, 127
directions, in qigong 37, 141
divinity 18, 82, 114, 138
dysmenorrhea 54

earth, connection to 19, 23, 24, 35, 46, 48, 50,
    82, 83, 94, 104, 106–7, 108
earth element 112–3, 115, 122, 123, 124, 129,
    131–2, 148
east, eastward 37, 116
emphysema 29
empty 26, 32, 34, 89, 134, 139, 140
ethics 19–20
equanimity 34
expand 32–3, 140
external 32, 33, 38, 141
eyes 18, 31, 38, 50, 53, 88, 116, 127, 132

fan zhe 37, 141
fang song gong 63, 146
fatigue 28, 133
finger exercise see nyasam
fire element 51, 112–3, 120–1, 123, 124, 129,
    131, 133
five elements 112–123, 131, 133
flesh 17, 24, 44, 122, 126
flexible 25, 41
fuel 21, 25, 27, 121, 133
full 32–4, 140

gallbladder 18, 80, 116
gallbladder meridian 51–2, 79–81, 113, 117,
    124, 126, 129
genitals 40, 117
gong 20–1
grandmother and grandchild, in five elements
    113, 131
Governor Vessel 40, 41, 50, 69

haemorrhoids 54
head hair 118
heart 18–20, 24, 25, 29, 31, 38, 42–3, 45, 48,
    51, 74, 119, 120–1, 132, 143, 146, 148
heart meridian 48–9, 55–59, 74, 113, 126,
    129, 130–1, 133
heat 51, 57, 74, 78, 86, 93, 120–1, 125, 126
heaven 18–19, 78,

herbalism 133
huangdi neijing 18
hun 18, 138–9
huqi, huxi 28, 140

idiom
    yong yi bu yong li 20, 139
    you yi, you qi, you li 20, 139
    ning jing zhi yuan 37, 141
    kuai ma jia bian 36, 141
    ma shang lai 30, 140
integrity 35, 126, 128
intention 19–20, 39, 75, 122
internal 32–3, 38, 141, 147
intimacy, intimate 32, 38, 51, 74

jing 17, 39, 118
joy 25, 33, 74, 120, 126
jue yin 130, 148

kidneys 17, 18, 41, 50, 65
kidney meridian 65–72
kong see empty
Kunlun mountains 65

large intestine 18, 113–4
large intestine meridian 53, 88–92, 113–4,
    127, 129
late summer 126–7
Larre, C. and Rochat de la Vallée, E. 19
legs, bringing qi to 107–111
li 20, 139
ligaments 116
linear 32, 37
lips 122
liver 18, 79–87
liver meridian 52, 54, 79–87
Luohan qigong 91, 147
lung meridian 52–3, 81–7, 114–5, 117, 127,
    129, 130, 131–2
lungs 17, 18, 29, 42, 44, 51–2, 81–7, 98, 105,
    114–5

mantra 13, 56
maturity 42, 120, 132
meditation 9, 96, 114, 115, 121, 128
metal element 112–5, 124, 129, 131, 139

Mitchell, S. 34, 136
moola, mula 40, 68
mother and child, in five elements 113, 123–4, 129, 131

nails 116
nature, the way of see fan zhe
neck injuries 65
nervous system 63–4
nipple line 53, 94
north, northward 37, 118
nyasam 97
palmar tendon 103–4
pairing meridians
    brothers and sisters 129
    harmonising dissonance 131–133
    six levels of energy 129–131
pectoral muscles 43, 49, 52, 105
pericardium 50
pericardium meridian 50–1, 73–5, 113, 120–1, 126, 129, 131
perineum 31, 40, 41, 45
po 18, 139
potential 33, 34, 36, 44, 68, 86
power 21, 41, 139
pranayama 28, 121
    see also breathing exercises
presence 34, 35, 126

qi, meaning energy 17–21
qi, meaning rise 35
qigong definition 20–1
radial tendon 51, 52, 103–4
rebound see fan zhe
relaxation 63, 90, 117, 121, 123, 128
    see also fang song gong
reserves 28, 44
restorative posture 71, 72, 89, 124, 128
rise, dynamic of movement 32, 35
root 22–3
ruo 37, 141

sacrum 41, 68, 95
sad, sadness 25, 74
sagittal suture 43
satisfaction 33–4, 122
seasonal transitions 123–8
sequencing see Index of Yoga Poses

shao yang 129–130
shao yin 129–131
shaolin 30, 138, 147
shen, meaning spirit 17–18, 39, 51
shibashi 46, 94, 98, 104, 108, 109, 144
shoulders injuries 65
shrink 32–3
sink 32, 35–6, 118
skin 114, 126, 132
skull, meridians on 42–3, 52
sleep 118
sleep medication 64
small intestine 120
small intestine meridian 49–50, 60–3, 113, 121, 126, 130
soft fist see zhang wo
solar plexus 51, 75
south, southward 37, 120
spinal disc injuries 65
spinal erectors 94
spiral 32–3, 38, 76
spirit see shen
spleen 18
spleen meridian 53–4, 79, 92–96
spring, springtime 22, 27, 116, 124–5
stability 119, 125, 132
sternum 43, 46
stomach 17, 18, 44, 51, 122
stomach meridian 53, 54, 92–96, 113, 129
strength 20–3, 33, 38, 39, 41–4, 86, 107, 117, 119
Strom, M. 20
summer 120, 125–7
superficial channels 48–49, 55, 88

tai yang 129–30, 148
tai yin 130, 148
Tao Te Ching 34, 136
tailbone 31, 40, 41, 45, 80, 89
tendons 17, 116, 125
third eye 43
thoracic spine 41, 71, 117
three yang 129–30
three yin 129–30
tiao xi 28
toil 21, 25, 27, 51
tongue 120
Torrent-Guasp, F. Dr 38
trajectory see linear

transition *see* Index of Yoga Poses
triple heater meridian 18, 51, 75–9, 113,
    120–1, 123, 126, 129

vacuum 34
vapours 21, 51
variations *see* Index of Yoga Poses
virtue 18–19, 20, 53
vital essence *see* jing

water 22, 23, 29, 34, 35, 38, 49, 50, 63, 67, 93,
    100, 102, 104, 107
water element 113, 117, 118, 121, 124, 128,
    129, 131–3
weakness *see* ruo
west, westward 37, 114
willpower 118–119
winter 27, 37, 118, 124, 128
wood element 112–3, 116–7, 124, 129, 131–2,
    138
wood coppicing 27

xing yi quan 98, 147
xiqi 28, 140

yang 40, 42, 129, 130, 133
Yang, J-M. Dr 28
yang meridians 129–30
yang ming 129, 148
yi, intention 20, 39
yin 40, 41
yin meridians 79, 129–30
yin yoga 63, 69, 128
yoga nidra 63, 119, 128
yoga, restorative 63
    see also restorative posture
yoga postures *see* sequencing

zhan zhuang 105, 147
zhang wo 86, 147
zhi 146
    see also willpower

INDEX OF EXERCISES

Bringing Qi to the Centre 94
Camel Pose Variation 70
Chair Pose and variations 80
Cloud Hands 101
Crane Arms 75
Deep Horse Stance 107
Dove Spreads Wings 82
Dragon Extends His Claws 99
Embrace the Void 105
Empty Stance 95, 123
Exhale to Close Fists 98
Expand to the Universe 105
Fisherman Casts His Net 102
Frontier Gates 73, 121
Funnel to the Earth 106, 123
Golden Rooster Shakes His Wings 56, 121
Great Eagle Spreads His Wings 90, 115
Gritted Teeth 89
Heel Drops 108
Holding Up the Sky 99, 108
Holy Crane Worships the Moon 109
Hook and Lift 103
Horse Breath 88, 115
Horse Stance 31
Kidney Recharge – Restorative Posture 72
Lion's Breath 88
Liver–Lung Exercises 1 to 4 83–86, 117
Macrocosmic Orbit 1 and 2 46–47
Microcosmic Orbit 41
Mischievous Boy Kicks His Leg 108

Nyasam 97
Old Monk Chops Wood 91, 117
Opening Shoulders and Arms 76
Opening to Earth 94, 115, 123
Opening to Heaven 81, 115
Pivot, Twist, Push 79, 117
Pressing Air 110
Pumping the Triple Heater 78, 123
Restorative Wrist Stretch 89
Rolling Ball 100, 121
Rolling the Qi Ball 92, 123
Separating Clouds 55
Sink Back 107
Small Intestine Exercise 1 and 2 61–62
Sparrowhawk Takes Flight 57
Sphinx Pose variation 69
Swimming Dragon variation 62
Three-Part Exhale 89
Waterfall – Restorative Posture 71, 119
Wild Goose: Cross Wings to Touch the
    Ground 66, 119
Wild Goose: Fly Over Water 67, 119
Wild Goose: Folding Nest 65, 119
Wild Goose: Opening Wings 65, 119
Wild Goose: Place Wings on Back 67, 119
Wild Goose: Shaking Wings 65, 119
Wrist Rolls 75

INDEX OF YOGA POSES FOR SEQUENCING, TRANSITIONS AND VARIATIONS

arm balances 57, 115, 119
Anuloma Viloma 21
Boat Pose 123
Bow Pose 121
Bridge Pose 115, 119, 121
Camel Pose 70, 115, 123
Chair Pose 48, 63, 80, 117
Child's Pose 64
Cobbler's Pose 95
Cobra Pose 115, 119, 121
Core work 94, 115, 126
Corpse Pose 64
Cow Facing Pose 95
Crescent Lunge 83, 117, 121
Crow Pose 63, 119
Dancer's Pose 107
Double Pigeon Pose 95
Downward Facing Corpse Pose 64
Downward Facing Dog Pose 76, 89, 115
Dropbacks 121
Eagle Pose 63, 84, 90, 107, 117
Easy Twist 87
Forearm Balance 117, 121
Forearm Plank Pose 117, 121
Flying Pigeon Pose 63
Garland Pose 95, 119

Gate Pose 123
Happy Baby Pose 64, 65, 117
Half Moon Pose 85, 107, 117
Handstand 86, 119, 121
Head to Knee Pose 95
Headstand 86, 117
Hero's Pose 61, 121
hip openers 94
hamstrings stretches 94
inversions 65, 70, 117, 128
Kapalabhati 121
Kneeling Warrior 87, 117
Knees to Chest Pose 115
Legs Up the Wall 64
Lizard Pose 119
Locust Pose 115, 119, 121, 123
meditation 96, 114, 115, 121, 127, 128
partner work 125–6
Pigeon Pose 95, 117
Plank Pose 76, 115, 117, 121
Plough Pose 64, 65, 119
Prayer Twist 87, 117
Pyramid Pose 61, 64, 78, 119
Revolving Triangle 87, 119
Seated Forward Fold 64
Seated Twist 117, 119, 121, 123

Seated Wide-Legged Forward Fold 64, 95, 117

Shoulderstand 64–5, 117, 119, 121

Side Angle Pose 82, 85, 115, 117

Side Crow Pose 63, 119

Side Plank Pose 115, 117, 121

Sphinx Pose 69–70, 119

standing balances 59, 70, 84, 107, 117, 119, 124

Standing Forward Fold 64–5, 117, 119

Standing Splits 119

Standing Wide-Legged Forward Fold 64, 86, 119

Supine Twist 115, 117, 119

Supported Splits 119

Sun Salutations 56, 59, 115, 117, 121, 123

Supported Shoulderstand 64–5, 119

Table Pose 121, 123

Temple Pose 48, 90, 121

Tree Pose 61, 75, 107, 117

Triangle Pose 82, 85, 117

Twisted Reverse Warrior 87

Twisting Half Moon 87, 119

Twisting Triangle *see* Revolving Triangle

Twisting Warrior 3 *see* Twisting Half Moon

Upward Facing Dog Pose 121

Warrior 1, 2 and 3 61, 82–4, 86, 91, 107, 117, 119

Wheel Pose 89, 121

Yoga Nidra 63, 119, 128

INDEX OF ACUPUNCTURE POINT NAMES IN ENGLISH

A Mound in the Wilderness 52, 145
Access Point to a Sea of Qi 67, 146
Access Point to the Kidneys 67, 146
Angled or Crooked Spring 43, 143
Binding Path 52, 145
Bright and Clear 52, 145
Bubbling or Original Spring 50, 144
Celestial or Heavenly Palace 53, 145
Central or Middle Pivot 41–2, 142
Centre of the Breast 95, 147
Correct or Upright Way of Being 52, 145
Crooked Spring 81, 147
Elevated Platform or Tower for the Spirit 42, 142
First or Original Mountain Pass 44, 144
Gateway of Clouds 53, 145
Gateway of Food Lubrication 93, 147
Gateway of Hope 52, 145
Gateway of Life 41, 119, 142
Gateway of Vitality 67–8, 146
Gateway to the Imperial City 43, 144
Gateway to the Yang Energy of the Loins 41, 142
Great Hammer 42, 142
Great Honesty or Esteem 52, 145
Hall of Impressions 42–3, 143

Heaven Rushes Out 43, 143
Heavenly Bone 78, 146
Heavenly Window 78, 147
Jade and Irregular Pearl 43, 143
Jade Hall or Court 43, 143
Lower Cavity or Duct 43, 144
Meeting of the Yin 41, 142
Middle Cavity or Duct 43, 144
One Hundred Meetings 42–3, 48, 143
Palace of Toil or Weariness 51, 55–8, 73, 95, 126, 144
Pathway of the Spirit 42, 142
Purple Palace 43, 143
Receiving of Broth or Fluid 43, 143
Residence of the Will or Hall of Ambition 67, 146
Sea of Blood 54, 146
Spring of Yang Energy 52, 145
Stone Gateway 44, 144
Sun and Moon 52, 145
Union of Valleys 53, 146
Upper Cavity or Duct 43, 144
Valiant or Heroic White 53, 145
Watchtower of the Spirit 43, 143
Wind Palace 42, 143
With the Full Force of Heaven 52, 144

CPI Antony Rowe
Eastbourne, UK
April 04, 2025